Assessment and Intervention with Children, Adolescents, and Adults with Neurocognitive Challenges

PSYCHODYNAMIC PSYCHOTHERAPY AND ASSESSMENT IN THE TWENTY-FIRST CENTURY

Series Editor

Steven Tuber, City University of New York at City College

Mission Statement

Psychodynamic Psychotherapy and Assessment establishes a milieu for the presentation of scholarly clinical work through a developmental lens. The emphasis throughout the series is on the integration of scholarship and practice through writings that are informed by both sources of learning. This domain includes works that document both evidence-based and traditional approaches within the field and applies these approaches to work with infants, children, adolescents, and adults. Efforts that link assessment to treatment are especially welcome, as are integrations between neuropsychological (brain-based) and psychological (mind or self-based) formulations about personality development and its aberrations. The impact of trauma, both chronic and acute, on the psychological lives of its victims is also an important area of study within this domain. New voices within the field are encouraged to write about the interface between the content and process of their emergent thinking and practice. In addition to the areas mentioned above, more experienced clinical scholars are encouraged to write about the supervisory process and its impact on both theory and practice. Works that focus on specific developmental processes and paradigms at points throughout the lifespan are another welcome area for contributions.

Titles in the Series

Assessment and Intervention with Children, Adolescents, and Adults with Neurocognitive Challenges: A Psychodynamic Perspective, by Nechama Sorscher

The Psychotherapy of Personality Disorders: Emergent Systems Theory as an Integrative Framework, by Lisa J. Cohen

Obsessive-Compulsive Disorder and Uncertainty: Struggling with a Shadow of a Doubt, by Moshe Marcus and Steven Tuber

Psychodynamics Commencing in Early Childhood: The Case for an Additional Tripartite Complex, by Joseph Newirth

Assessment and Intervention with Children, Adolescents, and Adults with Neurocognitive Challenges

A Psychodynamic Perspective

Nechama Sorscher

LEXINGTON BOOKS
Lanham • Boulder • New York • London

LEXINGTON BOOKS
Bloomsbury Publishing Inc, 1359 Broadway, New York, NY 10018, USA
Bloomsbury Publishing Plc, 50 Bedford Square, London, WC1B 3DP, UK
Bloomsbury Publishing Ireland, 29 Earlsfort Terrace, Dublin 2, D02 AY28, Ireland

BLOOMSBURY, ROWMAN & LITTLEFIELD and the ROWMAN & LITTLEFIELD logo are trademarks of Bloomsbury Publishing Plc

First published in the United States of America 2026

Cover design: Eleanor Rose
Cover photo © SLUSA Productions Savanna De Stefano

Library of Congress Cataloging-in-Publication Data
Names: Sorscher, Nechama, 1963– author.
Title: Assessment and intervention with children, adolescents, and adults with neurocognitive challenges : a psychodynamic perspective / Nechama Sorscher.
Description: Lanham : Lexington Books, [2024] | Series: Psychodynamic psychotherapy and assessment in the twenty-first century | Includes bibliographical references and index.
Identifiers: LCCN 2024013089 (print) | LCCN 2024013090 (ebook) | ISBN 9781666921687 (cloth) | ISBN 9781666921694 (epub)
Subjects: LCSH: People with disabilities. | Children with disabilities. | Autism—Diagnosis. | Attention-deficit hyperactivity disorder—Diagnosis.
Classification: LCC HV1568 .S6966 2024 (print) | LCC HV1568 (ebook) | DDC 362.4—dc23/eng/20240429
LC record available at https://lccn.loc.gov/2024013089
LC ebook record available at https://lccn.loc.gov/2024013090

ISBN: HB: 978-1-6669-2168-7
PB: 978-1-6669-2170-0
eBook: 978-1-6669-2169-4

Series: Psychodynamic Psychotherapy and Assessment in the Twenty-first Century

Typeset by Jones Ltd, London

For product safety related questions contact productsafety@bloomsbury.com.

To find out more about our authors and books visit www.bloomsbury.com and sign up for our newsletters.

This book is dedicated to my mentor and second mother,
Dr. Clarice Kestenbaum—whose guidance and love has been
instrumental in my journey as a therapist—and my amazing daughter
Rachel, who works harder than anyone I know.

Contents

Acknowledgments

First and foremost, I am deeply grateful to my patients and their families for allowing me the opportunity to enter their lives and appreciate their innermost struggles. It has been a profound gift and privilege to share with them the joys and challenges of living with neurocognitive disorders.

I gratefully acknowledge my colleague, Lisa Cohen, PhD, for her invaluable editing and critical feedback and my assistant, Alexander Celia, for his tireless hunting down of references—and for his support more generally. I'd also like to heartily thank Marsha Levy Warren, PhD, for being there at the beginning and for providing incisive supervision and boundless encouragement. Thank you to my parents, Esther and Yehuda Sorscher, for creating an intellectual and spiritual haven for me to flourish as a person and a professional. Lastly, I'd like to thank my late grandmother, Mamsie Yarmush, who was a beacon of light and love.

Acknowledgments

Chapter One

What Are Neurocognitive Challenges?

Neurocognitive challenges are remarkably prevalent. Nearly one in seven public school students receive special education services and one in 10 children are diagnosed with attention deficit hyperactivity disorder (ADHD) (CDC, 2019; National Center for Education Statistics, 2021). Nonetheless, these challenges are often misunderstood and misdiagnosed—both by the individuals manifesting these difficulties and by others. Neurodiversity and neurodivergence are the popular terms for describing individuals whose brains work differently than those of the majority of their peers. Neurodivergent children, adolescents, and adults demonstrate both learning and attention challenges that contribute to academic and social failures. Consequently, the socioemotional impact of these difficulties can be profound and may stretch well in adulthood. Many individuals with neurocognitive challenges will present for psychotherapy, complaining of depression, anxiety and low self-esteem; however, the link to their learning difficulties is not always obvious.

Recognizing the neurological underpinnings of these difficulties is a key element of psychotherapy with these individuals. Such recognition is essential for therapists if they are to gain an accurate portrait of their patients; communicating this understanding to them and thereby support their journey toward self-awareness and self-acceptance depends upon it. In addition, awareness of the neural pathways that underlie the neurocognitive impairments enhances therapists' ability to support the interventions and accommodations that may be necessary for these patients to function optimally.

Neurodivergence refers to the concept that is the cause of the learning, attentional, and/or social/emotional difficulties. These difficulties are neurocognitive in nature, and thus should be understood and treated from that perspective. Rather than attributing the individual's challenges to motivational or volitional roots, we must understand that the neural circuitry in the brain is functioning sub-optimally, resulting in mild to significant gaps in functioning. This insight is key when working with neurodivergent individuals—not just for psychologists, psychiatrists, and other counselors, but for the family members, educators, and employers of neurodivergent individuals. It is otherwise extremely common that the underlying neurobiological basis of these difficulties will be missed. Instead, such difficulties will be wrongly attributed to poor self-discipline, lack of motivation, lack of respect for the task, or generally low intelligence. Unsurprisingly, such misconceptions can have long lasting psychological effects. Moreover, they often lead to maladaptive coping mechanisms such as avoidance of relevant tasks and denial of one's difficulties, developed in response to the repeated experiences of failure and of "getting in trouble."

Neurocognitive disorders, such as learning and attention disorders and autism, are characterized by uneven neurocognitive development. Cognitive gaps may include deficits in basic academic skills, language development, or attention and memory. Depending on the area of impairment, an individual's scores on neuropsychological and neuroeducational testing batteries can range from Very Superior to Deficient. Importantly, individuals with specific neurocognitive difficulties often have normal overall intelligence; their deficits are select, not global. Likewise, different areas of the brain are compromised with different disorders: left hemisphere dysfunction in language-based disorders, right hemisphere impairment in visual-spatial disorders, frontal lobe dysfunction in attention deficits, and subcortical (as well as cortical) involvement in autism.

As noted above, these deficits have a far-reaching impact not only academically, but also emotionally and socially. Individuals with these disorders often incur repeated experiences of failure in both academic and social realms. The emotional consequences of these disorders include lowered self-esteem, pervasive feelings of shame, profound insecurity about academic skills, and a deep sense of vulnerability. In many cases, the resultant depression and anxiety symptoms are quite severe. Thus, many patients with neurocognitive difficulties will consult with psychotherapists for help in alleviating psychiatric symptoms. It is therefore essential that clinicians be mindful about the various types of learning disorders, understand their impact on the developing psyche, and be able to facilitate insight and awareness of these issues as well as adaptive responses to them. Clinicians can facilitate self-acceptance in their patients by highlighting the positive aspects of their challenge(s) and the unique adaptive qualities that each disorder brings.

WHAT ARE THE CAUSES OF NEUROCOGNITIVE CHALLENGES?

By definition, neurocognitive challenges are linked to atypical wiring in the brain. Learning disorders have a proven neurological base, as was initially found by examining the brains of patients with learning disabilities postmortem (Galaburda et al., 1985). Recent MRI and PET studies of children with neurocognitive challenges have confirmed that their brains work differently than neurotypical peers (Shaywitz & Shaywitz, 2005). People with nonverbal learning disorders have disordered functioning of the right hemisphere, the brain region that processes nonverbal information, including visual-spatial, intuitive, and organizational functions (Thompson, 1997). People with language-based disorders have reduced access to the left hemisphere of the brain, which underlies language-based tasks (Snowling, 200). Individuals with ADHD have reduced functioning of the prefrontal cortex, which mediates impulse control, planning and organization (Sowell et al., 2003). The most likely neurobiological base for autism is a widely distributed network of neural pathways on both a cortical and subcortical level; preliminary magnetic resonance spectroscopy findings confirm the presence of disruptions to these neural pathways (Katz et al., 2001).

Family studies of people with learning and attention disorders highlight the genetic contribution to these disabilities (Poelmans et al., 2011). In addition, exposure to toxins such as mercury, either in utero or during childhood, is another possible contributing factor (Martin et al., 2000, Morrow et al., 2006). Low birthweight is also associated with development of learning disorders (Aarnoudse-Moens et al., 2009). Further, the interpersonal environment has a significant impact on brain development; under stimulation, in particular, can strongly compromise children's cognitive abilities.

CATEGORIES OF NEUROCOGNITIVE CHALLENGE

DSM-5 TR lists eight categories under neurodevelopmental disorders. These are: intellectual disorders, communication disorders, autism spectrum disorder, attention-deficit/hyperactivity disorder, specific learning disorders, motor disorders, tic disorders, and other neurodevelopmental disorders.

The three most common categories of neurocognitive challenges, however, are: learning disorders, attention disorders, and high functioning autism. As these are the disorders most likely to be seen in clinical practice, we will restrict our discussion in this book to these three categories.

Further, because these disorders are generally studied within a developmental framework, most of the relevant research is performed on children; therefore, we will mostly refer to children in this part of the discussion. However, adolescents and adults also struggle with these challenges, as will be addressed throughout the book. It should be noted that there is overlap between the categories and many individuals suffer from both attention and learning disorders. However, for the sake of clarity, I will discuss each diagnostic category as a single entity.

LEARNING DISORDERS

Silver (2006) broke down the learning process into four components: input (getting information into the brain), integration (making sense of the information), memory (storage and retrieval of information), and output (the physical response, such as speech or motor activity). A learning disorder can be manifested at any stage of this process.

Language-Based Disorders

Most learning disorders can be grouped into two major areas, language-based and visual-spatial learning disorders. Patients with language-based learning disorders present with relatively weak language skills and stronger visual-spatial skills. Language disorders are divided into receptive and expressive spheres. With receptive disorders, children have difficulty processing auditory information, following directions, and understanding verbal and written content. With expressive disorders, children present with diminished vocabulary, poor syntax and grammar, faulty oral and written expression, and poor organization, both in speech and writing.

Receptive Language Disorders

Children with receptive language disorders have trouble at the input level, as reflected in their lack of comprehension of material. They have difficulty following directions, understanding academic information, and making sense of social situations. They often demonstrate dysfluent speech and a diminished vocabulary. These children are at greater risk for academic and social failure due to this significant deficiency. Children with receptive language disorders may also have an auditory processing disorder, though auditory processing disorder is a more general deficit stemming from poor processing of auditory information. However, once the child processes the information, comprehension is often intact to superior. In contrast, receptive language disorder stems from a specific deficit in how the child comprehends words on a neurocognitive level.

Auditory Processing Disorder

Auditory processing deficits, though not strictly a language-based disorder, often co-occur with receptive language disorders. These disorders also occur at the input level; children have difficulty making sense of the auditory information that is presented to them. These challenges are not due to hearing issues at the level of the ear, though they are related to the way the brain takes in the auditory information. These children mishear information or simply do not register that information is being directed at them. They are often noise sensitive and may present with slurred or unintelligible speech. They have a great deal of difficulty focusing on a noisy environment. Often, they do not understand rapid or accented speech. These deficits pose significant challenges in the classroom, at home and on the playground (Geffner and Swain et al., 2007). Let us consider a case example:

Charlotte, a vivacious 6-year-old girl with sparkling blue eyes, presented as a behavioral enigma to her parents and teachers. Although clearly bright and a precocious reader, Charlotte preferred to spend the majority of her time in the classroom sitting in the book corner, shielding herself with soft pillows and refusing to participate in classroom activities. Her parents commented that, at home, she was an engaging girl who, while shy and reserved with peers, played nicely with her younger sister and was very cooperative with her parents. Neuropsychological assessment revealed a significant auditory processing disorder; her avoidant behavior in the classroom was the result of her compromised language processing skills. Overwhelmed by the noise, she preferred to avoid activities and sit by herself in a quiet corner. In addition, she did not understand the directions for activities and thus could not comply with tasks and routines. Charlotte's classroom was outfitted with a system that allowed her to clearly hear the teachers' instructions. She was also provided with speech and language therapy. Within a few months, Charlotte joined her peers during school activities and was able to progress academically and socially.

Expressive Language Disorders

Children with expressive language disorders have difficulties on the output level. Such children have excellent comprehension but impaired speech production. Their speech is halting and dysfluent, and they often jumble the order of sentences while using poor syntax and grammar. These children demonstrate significant word retrieval difficulties, such as the "tip of the tongue" phenomenon, when they cannot find the correct word that they are seeking. They may stammer and hesitate and fill their speech with words such as "umm" and "uh" in an attempt to express themselves. Although their receptive vocabulary is excellent and they understand conversations, they often cannot participate in them as they become tongue tied and the words do not come out correctly. Thus, they can become very frustrated as they cannot communicate their ideas or understanding of a situation effectively.

Nonverbal Learning Disorder

Individuals with nonverbal learning disabilities often present with strong language skills and weak visual-spatial skills. Visual processing (input) is often impaired. Children with visual processing difficulties may demonstrate impaired depth perception, misperception or rotation of numbers and letters, and poor visual-motor skills, as when catching a ball or completing puzzles. In addition, graphomotor skills are often compromised as the child cannot copy letters or adequately perform pencil and paper tasks. Visual memory is often deficient as well and the child presents with an extremely poor sense of direction. The child also has difficulty with visual-spatial alignment and any tasks that require a sense of spatial awareness. Thus, visual sequencing in math is incredibly difficult for the child; organizing papers, managing time, and keeping one's belongings orderly all present significant challenges.

As they develop academically, these children may learn to compensate for their visual-spatial issues in reading and writing with their strong language skills—but may struggle in math and science, as these subjects are more dependent on visual information. In addition, as their visual memory is often compromised, they have great difficulty retaining numerical facts. They often work slowly due to impaired visual efficiency, and they fatigue quickly, as processing visual information is laborious for them. Oftentimes writing can also be a struggle due to their difficulties with organizing and sequencing. Reading speed can also be compromised by poor visual processing, making reading a laborious and frustrating task. As noted above, visual sequencing skills are often deficient. Thus, the child has difficulty complying with tasks that require visual sequencing, such as standing in an orderly line with classmates or finding the correct page in a book.

Thompson (1996) enumerates the characteristics of the nonverbal learning-disabled student and describes a child at risk for academic, social, and emotional failures. She explains that, because their right hemisphere systems are dysfunctional, these children are rigid and have difficulty with transitions.

Significant visual-spatial and motoric challenges result in a compromised sense of direction, sloppy handwriting, and difficulty learning gross motor activities, such as riding a bike. There is also impaired awareness of social nuances, as interpersonal skills are often mediated by visual-spatial processes, such as attention to facial cues and body language. The following is a case example of a nonverbal learning disorder:

> Leslie was a vibrant young graduate student in public history at a competitive institution. Although she could easily understand the material and concepts in class and had excellent reading comprehension, she struggled in her program to complete her assignments. In addition, personal hygiene and the cleanliness of her room were ongoing areas of difficulty for her, and led to great shame. Further, she had trouble connecting with her classmates and expressed that they were all more advanced and academically "together" than her. Therapy helped her recognize that all these challenges were a direct result of her nonverbal learning disorder.

On a positive note, individuals with nonverbal learning disorder tend to be excellent readers and are often highly verbal and articulate. Professions that have an emphasis on reading and writing are well suited for them, and these individuals can function well as professors, researchers (especially in the social science realm), editors, and lawyers.

Both language-based learning disorders and nonverbal learning disorders are often comorbid with more specific academic disorders in reading, writing and math. These disorders will be reviewed below.

Reading Disorders

Broadly defined, dyslexia refers to difficulty reading. Children with dyslexia demonstrate poor reading fluency, impaired reading accuracy, and deficient reading comprehension. They typically present early with letter reversals, impoverished sight vocabulary (the number of written words they recognize automatically), and dysfluency, that is, a choppy reading style. These challenges partially arise from visual processing impairments and are then compounded by language-based deficits and weak working memory (Pennington & Bishop, 2009). Working memory involves the mental manipulation of information—more specifically the ability to hold information in the mind and use it in the execution of cognitive tasks. Our working memory holds new information in consciousness so the brain can work with it in real time and integrate it with other information. As reading depends on the ability to recognize words, to build up a sight vocabulary, and to make connections between words, a poor working memory interferes with acquiring these skills. Sarah offers an illustration of dyslexia:

> Sarah, a sensitive, empathetic 7-year-old girl loved to look at books and seemed to enjoy reading them. However, her phonics skills (i.e., the ability to match sound with symbol in letter identification) were exceptionally low and her sight word vocabulary was very poor. In time, her mother realized that Sarah was memorizing the books in school as they were read to her and that her "reading" was actually pure memorization. A neuropsychological evaluation revealed severe dyslexia. She was referred for Orton-Gillingham instruction, a specialized, data-based remediation geared at improving her phonics skills. As a result, her reading improved, although she continues to present with choppy, dysfluent, and slow reading skills.

Although visual processing issues play a role, language-based learning disabilities make up the majority of dyslexic disorders, as reading is fundamentally about decoding and comprehending words. Children who know how to decode but evidence significant comprehension difficulties often demonstrate language deficits along with poor abstract reasoning skills. For example, a child may read a paragraph fluently but have little idea of its meaning, and so will be unable to answer related questions appropriately. In addition, these learners often suffer from poor working memory, so they have great difficulty with building up their sight vocabulary, retaining non-contextual information (as in a list of unrelated words), and recalling the details of a story. Each of these reading skills are dependent on the ability to hold information in your mind while attending to tasks.

It is important to note that there are positive aspects of having dyslexia. For example, individuals with dyslexia tend to see the world in a visual manner and are often quite artistic and creative. Visual-spatial thinkers see patterns and can come up with ideas that are innovative and exciting. For example, artists, designers, inventors, and architects all work in professions that benefit from visual-spatial thinking.

Written Expressive Disorder

Written expression impairment is another byproduct of language-based learning disorders, as writing is another academic skill that primarily depends on facility with words. Children may have difficulty organizing their writing, using proper grammar and syntax, coming up with evocative words, and supporting their ideas with sufficient detail. Children may also have graphomotor difficulties, rendering their handwriting sloppy and laborious. In the classroom, these learners are at a disadvantage as they may have difficulty following directions, participating in class, retaining information, taking notes, and producing content in class, on homework, and on tests. Notably, difficulties with written expression and following classroom rules and expectations commonly co-occur with all of the learning disorders mentioned above—that is, nonverbal and other language-based learning disorders.

Math Disorders

Dyscalculia is a deficit in the ability to perform math-related tasks. Children can present with impaired numerical computation skills, difficulty recalling math facts, poor ability to set up algorithms, and inefficient computation skills. Dyscalculia can stem from different learning disorders. Children with language-based disorders may have particular difficulty with word problems. Children with impaired working memory have difficulty retaining numerical facts and manipulating them in their mind. Poor abstract reasoning skills lead to difficulty setting up problems and applying algorithms. Children with nonverbal learning disorders, however, are typically weaker in math and science due to their visual-spatial processing deficits, as numerical capacity is associated with spatial abilities and sense of pattern and design.

ATTENTION DEFICIT HYPERACTIVITY DISORDER

We will now turn to the second category of neurocognitive disorder addressed in this book, ADHD. Gensler (2011) delineated attention as an executive function that helps a person process information effectively, narrow down options, and make decisions. People with attentional difficulties frequently have abnormalities in their reticular activation systems or the posterior cortical areas, rendering them distractible, impulsive, and inefficient with processing information. In 1972, Douglas (1972) described a set of characteristics that then became widely known as attention deficit disorder or ADD. Barkley (1990) wrote the seminal book entitled *Attention Deficit Hyperactivity Disorder (ADHD)*, delineating the characteristics of both ADD and ADHD. Currently, specific DSM 5-TR diagnoses include ADHD with three subtypes; predominantly inattentive, predominantly hyperactive-impulsive, and combined (American Psychiatric Association, 2022). However, Ratey (1994) suggested that the concept of attention deficit is imprecise and that this disorder is better understood as attention inconsistency, the inability to sustain attention or flexibly allocate it rather than to attend at all.

The diagnostic criteria for inattention are that the individual fails to give close attention to details, has difficulty sustaining attention in tasks, does not seem to listen when spoken to, does not follow through on instructions, and fails to finish schoolwork, chores or duties in the workplace. Criteria for hyperactivity include demonstrating fidgety behavior, running about, being often on the go, and appearing "driven by a motor." Impulsivity is demonstrated by such behavior as blurting out answers, having difficulty awaiting turns, and interrupting or intruding on others. Let us consider a case example:

> Noah, a serious 8-year-old boy, was referred by his mother for an assessment due to school-related difficulties. Although Noah was engaged in class and participated with meaningful comments, he had great difficulty completing assignments on time. His backpack and desk were messy and disorganized. Most telling was his teacher's observation that she would hand Noah a paper and, from the time it took for him to walk from her desk back to his seat, he would lose it. Testing revealed a diagnosis of ADHD, Inattentive Type.

Children with ADHD frequently exhibit impaired executive functioning along with inattentiveness and poor inhibitory control (Conway, 2014). They often fatigue easily and may experience difficulty with completing assignments. Further, they demonstrate cognitive rigidity and have severe difficulty negotiating transitions, shifting mindsets, and adapting to complicated and novel situations.

Children and adults with ADHD may also demonstrate significant social/emotional difficulties. They can have poor affect regulation and can get overly excited and happy, as well as depressed and discouraged. Their frustration tolerance can be exceedingly low as they easily give up when presented with challenges, become anxious and avoidant, and can even be explosive, such that they throw tantrums, cry, and become aggressive (although such temper tantrums are more common in children than adults). Both adults and children can be socially intrusive as they are impulsive, lack a "filter," and can be needy and demanding in interpersonal relations. It should be noted, however, that many adults with ADD mature and develop compensatory strategies that alleviate these social issues. Nonetheless, there are adults who still struggle with these symptoms.

Neuroimaging studies have highlighted the areas of the brain most affected by this disorder. MRI studies document abnormalities in the prefrontal cortex, the part of the brain responsible for decision making and planning; the corpus callosum, which transfers information from one hemisphere of the brain to another; and the caudate nucleus, which is involved with memory and motor inhibition (Shaw et al., 2006). Further, abnormalities in cortical thickness, that is, delays in cortical maturation, were also found, although ADHD children caught up with their neurotypical peers over time in this regard (Gopin & Healey, 2014). As with learning disorders, there is a strong genetic/familial influence. Exposure to toxins, both in utero and during development, is also a risk factor for the development of ADHD (Fried, et al., 1997).

It is important to note that there are positive aspects of ADHD. Individuals with ADHD are often uniquely poised to navigate our current culture as their attention span is quite flexible. They are able to "hyperfocus" on tasks that catch their interest and so can happily spend hours on creative pursuits, computer programming, or other areas of interest. They also tend to retain a childlike playfulness, spontaneity, imagination, and sense of wonder. These qualities are essential to many creative and scientific pursuits. Their extraordinarily high level of energy and "roaming" quality of attention, that is, they can notice many details simultaneously, can contribute to productivity and the ability to juggle tasks. A partial list of occupations that suit individuals with ADHD includes entrepreneurs, salespeople, inventors, artists, and fitness instructors.

AUTISM SPECTRUM DISORDER

Autism Spectrum Disorder (ASD) is the third category of neurocognitive disorder that we will address in this book. ASD has garnered increasing attention in the media, and there is evidence that it has become more frequently diagnosed in recent decades (Christensen, et al., 2019). Autism spectrum disorder is characterized by deficits in multiple areas of development, including social relations, communication, and a range of interests and activities. Individuals with autism have difficulty socializing with peers and communicating appropriately. They typically do not understand their own feelings or other people's feelings, and are markedly ill-attuned to social dynamics. They are often preoccupied with a rigid range of interests and activities and engage in restrictive, repetitive, and stereotypical behaviors. Additionally, they can become quite agitated when their routines are disrupted, or when they face moments of overstimulation. While their academic difficulties are more variable, they can present with poor working memory along with impaired selective attention and complex information processing. The most likely neurobiological basis for autism involves abnormalities across a network of subcortical and cortical structures (Katz, Goldstein & Beers, 2001). The following case example illustrates a number of these traits:

Matt, a bespectacled and "geeky" 12-year-old boy, was in the eighth grade at a competitive private school. Although he was holding his own academically, he presented with significant social difficulties. Of note, he spoke in a monotone, maintained poor eye contact, and tended to go into excruciating detail when telling anecdotes. He was obsessed with transportation and had an encyclopedic retention of any facts related to trains, planes, and cars, which he would recite pedantically with little attention to his companion's level of interest. These social/interpersonal deficits are typical of individuals with high-functioning autism.

According to DSM-5-TR, to meet diagnostic criteria for autism spectrum disorder, an individual must have persistent deficits in social communication and interaction as well as restrictive, repetitive behaviors. Impaired social relations would include poor social or emotional reciprocity. Children with this disorder demonstrate deficits in developing, maintaining, and understanding peer relationships and engaging in developmentally appropriate play.

Communication deficits are described as difficulty sustaining a conversation as well as a tendency toward stereotyped language. For example, autistic individuals may repeat words or sentences, quote extensively from movies or TV shows, or repeat the same ideas in a conversation. In addition, they demonstrate deficits in nonverbal communicative behaviors used for social interaction, for example with abnormalities in eye contact and body language. Lastly, preoccupation with objects, parts of objects, and specific areas of interest along with inflexible adherence to routines and rituals are hallmarks of this disorder. Concomitantly, hyper- or hypo-reactivity to sensory input or unusual interest in sensory aspects of the environment can also manifest. They may be overly sensitive to texture, for example, and unable to wear itchy clothing. Concomitantly, they may have impaired pain perception and even engage in self-injurious behaviors without feeling pain.

Individuals with high-functioning autism demonstrate cognitive deficits in various domains at the complex (but not simple) skill level. Notably, they have significant difficulty with recognizing the gestalt, and tend to overly focus on tangential details—a tendency that compromises them both academically and socially. Their working memory is often poor due to their seizing on irrelevant details and missing the point of a story, conversation, or lecture. Thus, they present as concrete and rigid and unable to cope with complex, abstract information unless it is presented in a highly-structured manner. In sum, autistic individuals process the world as it consists of details but cannot easily organize the details into an integrated whole. Instead, they may use a laborious, logical sequencing of information that can be accurate and precise but is time consuming and therefore not efficient.

Individuals on the spectrum may have difficulty identifying feelings, empathizing with others, and engaging socially. They cannot intuit social gestalts or emotional nuances because they do not process emotional states holistically. Additionally, they can become easily agitated and overloaded as they have low tolerance for disruption to their routine or any type of sensory stimulation, such as noise, lights, or crowds. This agitation has a neurocognitive basis as they lack pattern recognition and holistic thinking, which allows for rapid albeit general processing of large amounts of information. Thus, large amounts of new information presented at once can overwhelm them. Such individuals can process a good deal of information if presented in a sequential manner, but they require chunking of information to recognize the gestalt.

Nonetheless, individuals with autism may have the capacity for intense attentional focus and to commit large amounts of factual information to memory, if not always to synthesize it into a coherent whole. When learning to read, children with autism may also present with hyperlexia; that is, they can read fluently—often at a precocious age—but cannot comprehend the material. Autistic individuals often develop significant expertise in one area, for example science, transportation, or baseball facts, and can appear as a savant within this area. This expertise reflects their capacity for hyper-focused attention and their ability to remember large amounts of factual information. However, they may then present with deficits in areas in which they lack basic skills or do not have interest.

As with many other neurodivergent conditions, there are benefits to ASD. Individuals with ASD are incredibly attuned to details and are able to perform obsessive, detail-oriented work that other people would see as boring and tedious. In addition, as they are often visual-spatial learners and can solve complicated problems using that type of reasoning. Jobs that are suited for individuals with autism spectrum disorder include engineers, computer programmers, accountants, army intelligence and lab technicians.

In sum, neurocognitive challenges are prevalent among children, adolescents, and young adults. These deficits have a far-reaching impact, academically, socially, and emotionally. Because of this, individuals with neurocognitive challenges are particularly susceptible to depression, anxiety, low self-esteem and intense feelings of shame and anxiety. Thus, they will frequently consult with therapists to help them with the social-emotional sequelae of these disorders. It is therefore imperative for clinicians to acquire some basic understanding of these diagnostic categories as effective intervention must take into account both the neurocognitive and psychiatric challenges that they face. When working with patients with neurocognitive challenges, being aware of their strengths and helping them identify and celebrate their areas of strength can be crucial to improving self-esteem, reducing depression and anxiety, and setting them up for academic, social, and occupational success. The following chapters will address assessment and intervention with this population.

Chapter Two

How to Evaluate Neurocognitive Challenges

Patients with neurocognitive difficulties are typically referred to neuropsychologists for a comprehensive assessment in order to determine cognitive strengths and deficits. A neuropsychological evaluation can be invaluable in helping diagnose the patient, recommending services and accommodations, and facilitating self-awareness. With children, it can also help parents and teachers better understand the child. A comprehensive assessment is critical in establishing the etiology of deficits, as learning and attention difficulties may stem from many causes. They can have a psychiatric origin (e.g., depression or psychosis) or a neurological source (such as seizures or dementia). Alternatively, such deficits may have a neurocognitive etiology, reflecting impaired functioning or inadequate development in that part of the brain responsible for those skills. The assessment rules out different possibilities and confirms an accurate diagnosis. This chapter will elucidate the fundamentals of assessment, review best testing practices, and give examples of test reports.

A typical neuropsychological battery covers several neurocognitive domains, including general intelligence, academic achievement, speech and language, attention, memory, auditory processing, visuo-spatial processing, and motor skills. A personality section is often included to provide insight into any relevant emotional issues, including self-esteem, anxiety, depression, and other aspects of social/emotional functioning. The report carefully details the nuances of the patient's challenges and strengths. Best testing practices include a detailed background section that encompasses development, family history, social/emotional/academic functioning, and medical history. In addition, a careful analysis of all neurocognitive domains is detailed in the report. Further, behavioral observations should be provided to convey the patient's functioning during the testing process.

CHOOSING THE TESTS

Selecting a test battery is specific to the patient; however, there is a core battery of tests that provides basic information on cognitive functioning. The evaluator can then add on tests that are more tailored to the individual. Although it is beyond the scope of this chapter to describe each test in detail, I will briefly describe some of the most frequently used or representative tests below.

The Wechsler IQ tests are widely used as a baseline of performance, a screening of potential challenges, and an overall measure of academic potential. David Wechsler developed this test to assess intelligence in a practical and clinical way (Thambirajah and Ramanujan, 2016). The Wechsler Intelligence Scale for Children is currently in its fifth edition (WISC-V; Wechsler, 2014) while the Wechsler Adult Intelligence Scale is in its fourth edition (WAIS-IV; Wechsler, 2014). WISC and WAIS scores have been correlated with academic achievement; both tests generate a multi-test score profile that illuminates the person's learning style. The IQ scores are separated into four indices: Verbal, Visual-Spatial, Working Memory, and Processing Speed. Each index reveals valuable information that is age-normed so the individual's performance can be compared with that of his or her same-aged peers.

While the WAIS and WISC measure cognitive function, they are not intended to assess academic performance. Instead, a wide variety of academic skills-based tests are available and frequently used. The Wechsler Individual Achievement Test–4th Edition (WIAT-4; Wechsler, 2020) is coordinated with the Wechsler IQ tests so the evaluator can obtain a standardized achievement score that is statistically comparable with the IQ scores. This is important, as a large discrepancy between intellectual ability and academic performance is often indicative of a learning disability. The WIAT assesses a wide range of academic skills, including reading accuracy, reading comprehension, numerical facility, spelling, and written expression. However, the WIAT's assessment of academic skills can be cursory in nature, and there are other academic tests that are more detailed or focused, such as the Grey Oral Reading Test–Fifth Edition (GORT-5, Bryant, 2012). The GORT-5 evaluates reading accuracy, fluency, and comprehension with multi-sentence paragraphs. The Test of Written Language (TOWL, Hammil & Larsen, 1996) scores writing on diverse criteria, including organization and theme development.

There is also a plethora of speech and language tests, ranging from a quick and superficial assessment of receptive and expressive language, such as the Peabody Expressive and Receptive Test (Gardner, 2000), which assesses the individual's ability to either name pictures (expressive) or indicate understanding of a word by pointing to one out of four pictures that best describes the word (receptive). The Clinical Evaluation of Language Fundamentals–Fifth Edition (CELF-5, Semel et al., 2013) is more nuanced and comprehensive. The CELF is widely used, as it assesses diverse speech and language skills, such as sentence structure, syntax, grammar, auditory memory, and word definition skills.

Memory provides another domain of assessment. Memory is a complicated construct that requires careful assessment with varied memory tests, such as the Wide Range Assessment of Memory and Learning–Third Edition (WRAML; Adams & Sheslow, 2021) and the Wechsler Memory Scales- IV (WMS-IV; Wechsler, 2009). Both visual and auditory memory are assessed on these tests.

Attention is a crucial multidimensional construct that is vital to assess, as it contributes significantly to academic success. Attention, which broadly means the ability to maintain focus on a particular task, encompasses a range of neurocognitive skills, such as impulse control, resistance to distraction, and ability to execute transitions. Thus, attention can be difficult to assess and requires multiple assessment measures. The Continuous Performance Test (CPT; Connors, 1995) is the "gold standard" of attention tests. It is a test of vigilance that requires attention to a visual or auditory presentation of randomly occurring letters and asks the participant to either respond or inhibit a response to the letters. For example, a participant is instructed to press the space bar after all letters except the letter X. Processing speed, sustained attention, ability to inhibit inaccurate responses, and execute transitions flexibly are all measured. Two others widely used tests include the Stroop Color and Word Test (SCWT; Stroop, 1935), a brief measure of selective or focused attention, and the Wisconsin Card Sorting Test (WCST; Heaton, 1981) a measure of cognitive flexibility, or the ability to shift tasks efficiently. The Delis-Kaplan Executive Function System evaluates higher level cognitive skills, specifically nonverbal and verbal executive functioning skills (DKEFS; Kaplan & Kramer, 20001).

Several tests are used to evaluate motor skills. Graphomotor functioning is assessed with the Developmental Test of Visual Motor Integration (VMI, Fourth Edition; Beery, 1997), which requires the patient to copy designs, and the Bender-Gestalt Test, which evaluates both the quality and the placement of the designs copied from images of geometric figures (Bender, 1946). The Purdue Pegboard measures finger dexterity and has been shown to discriminate between children with and without learning disabilities (Kane & Gill, 1972).

Auditory processing is assessed with the SCAN-C Test for Auditory Processing in Children (SCAN-C, 3, Keith, 1994). This test provides four scores on subtests tapping auditory attention and auditory discrimination in both ears. For example, competing words are piped into both ears and clients are asked to say the word that they heard in their right ear.

When autism is suspected, the Autism Diagnostic Observation Schedule-2 (ADOS) can be administered (ADOS-2, Gotham et al., 2006). This test assesses social and communicative behaviors relevant to an autism diagnosis. The Behavior Assessment System for Children (BASC-3, Reynolds & Kamphaus, 2020) is also administered to screen for general social/emotional problems; although the test is not specific to autism, its findings can help with determining an autism diagnosis. This is a questionnaire for parents and teachers to complete that is then scored across different domains, such as attentional, social, somatic and other behavioral realms. In addition, the Social Responsiveness Scale—Second Edition (SARS-2) identifies the presence and severity of social impairment characteristic of individuals within the autism spectrum (Constantino and Gruber, 2012).

Finally, personality traits that might contribute to or provide context for the individual's learning challenge are typically assessed with projective tests. Projective tests present the individual with ambiguous stimuli, such as inkblots, which encourage the test taker to project his or her feelings onto the pictures. The benefit of projective tests is their relative protection from self-report biases as it is difficult for patients to understand what kind of information they are disclosing. Data from the Rorschach (Rorschach, 1942) and the Thematic Apperception Test (TAT; Murray, 1943) are used to elucidate any psychiatric issues such as anxiety, depression, or psychotic thought process. The responses also provide information about defensive style, judgment, impulse control, self-esteem, sociability and other personality variables. While the TAT is scored qualitatively–no normed scoring systems are widely used, the Rorschach has two normed and evidence-based scoring systems, the Exner Comprehensive Scoring System (Exner, 1993) and the Rorschach Performance Assessment System (R-PAS; Meyer, Viglione, Mihura, Erard, & Erdberg, 2011).

The above tests represent a personal core battery that can be adapted to the individual by adding or subtracting tests as needed.

TEST REPORT EXAMPLES

We will now review excerpts from test reports assessing individuals with each disorder discussed in Chapter 1 to illustrate their typical neuropsychological profiles.

Language-Based Learning Disorder

Individuals with language-based learning disorders demonstrate relatively weaker verbal skills as compared with visual-spatial skills. This discrepancy is present on the IQ tests, memory tasks, and specific language tests. Typically, these patients will also demonstrate disorders in reading and expressive writing as these skills are language-based. I will now present an excerpt from a report of a child with speech and language delays. I am only including those sections that highlight his language delays.

Michael was an 8-year-old boy who was referred by his mother due to concerns about poor academic performance. As can be seen from the excerpt, poor performance on the language-based tasks confirm the presence of a language-based learning disability and illustrates the need for accommodations and intervention. Michael's scores on the CELF-4 are in Table 2.1.

Michael's basic language abilities were assessed with the Clinical Evaluation of Language Fundamentals—Fourth Edition (CELF-4). Language processing skills refer to a child's ability to "take in" information that is presented through language (receptive language) and to use language to express his understanding of an idea (expressive language). According to his performance on the CELF-4, Michael's core language skills, which include both expressive and receptive language abilities, fall in the Profoundly Impaired range, at the 0.1st percentile.

Table 2.1. Clinical Evaluation of Language Fundamentals—Fourth Edition (CELF-4): Michael

Indices	*SS*	*Percentile*	*Qualitative Rating*
Core Language	52	0.1st	Profoundly Impaired
Receptive Language	73	4th	Borderline
Expressive Language	53	0.1st	Profoundly Impaired
Language Content	78	7th	Borderline
Language Memory	47	<0.1st	Profoundly Impaired
Subtest	*SS*	*Percentile*	*Qualitative Rating*
Concepts & Following Directions	2	0.4th	Profoundly Impaired
Recalling Sentences	1	0.1st	Profoundly Impaired
Formulated Sentences	1	0.1st	Profoundly Impaired
Word Classes—Receptive	8	25th	Average
Word Classes—Expressive	5	5th	Borderline
Word Classes—Total	6	9th	Low Average
Word Definitions	9	37th	Average
Understanding Spoken Paragraphs	4	2nd	Borderline

Michael's performance on the CELF-4's Receptive Language Index suggests uneven skill development in the areas of comprehension and listening. On a task in which he was asked to point to pictures of objects in response to oral directions, Michael was not able to interpret, recall, and execute complex oral commands (0.4th percentile). He struggled with multi-step directions and his performance within the subtest was uneven, correctly executing harder items while missing some easier ones. Nonetheless, Michael's score on a task that tapped capacity to understand relationships between words was adequate (25th percentile); for example, he understood how a "circle and a square go together." This relative area of strength is consistent with his earlier performance on the WISC-V in which he displayed the ability to recognize categories. For example, he correctly said that "a table and a chair are both furniture." Thus, some regions of receptive language are intact.

The CELF 4's Expressive Language Index is a cumulative measure of Michael's performance on subtests that probe expressive aspects of language, including oral language expression. His expressive language abilities fall within the Profoundly Impaired range (0.1st percentile). He struggled on all subtests, which included tasks that required him to complete orally presented sentences that pertain to an illustration; for example, when presented with a picture of children sitting around a table and asked to describe the picture he said "children" but could not describe the activity. He was similarly unable to formulate sentences using target words or phrases and to imitate sentences presented by the examiner.

In sum, Michael displayed significant weaknesses in his expressive and receptive language processing skills throughout the CELF-4. His performance corresponds with earlier evaluations, which revealed delays in language processing. As such, it was recommended that Michael should continue with intense speech and language intervention.

Dyslexia

Dyslexia is a specific reading disorder that is diagnosed when the child's reading skills fall significantly below average. In addition, phonemic awareness, that is, the ability to execute sound-symbol association, is often deficient. Phonemic awareness is one of the key components of learning how to read (Shaywitz & Shaywitz, 2005). Visual-spatial challenges may also be detected, such as letter reversals (Mather & Wendling, 2011).

This excerpt illustrates the typical performance of a child with dyslexia. More specifically, we can see the impact of compromised visual and auditory processing skills on reading acquisition. Sally is a 6-year-old girl who was

Table 2.2. Wechsler Individual Achievement Test—Third Edition (WIAT-III) and NEPSY-II: Sally

WIAT-III			
Subtest	*SS*	*Percentile*	*Qualitative Rating*
Early Reading Skills	91	27th	Average
Word Reading	88	21st	Average
Pseudoword Decoding	84	14th	Average
Basic Reading Composite	**86**	**18th**	**Average**
Numerical Operations	83	13th	Below Average
Math Problem Solving	109	73rd	Average
Mathematics	**95**	**37th**	**Average**
Alphabet Writing Fluency	94	34th	Average
Spelling	84	14th	Below Average
NEPSY-II			
Subtest	*SS*	*Percentile*	*Qualitative Rating*
Phonological Processing	9	37th	At Expected Level

referred to testing by her mother due to concerns about acquiring reading skills. Her mother noted that she loves books and memorizes the words but has not yet acquired letter-sound recognition. Her scores on the WIAT-III are presented in Table 2.2.

Sally's performance on standardized achievement measures was variable and ranged from Below Average to Average. Using age-based norms on the WIAT-III, Sally's basic reading skills fell at the low end of the Average range for her age. She was able to identify most letters (although she reversed "b" and "d"), letter sounds, and rhyming words, and to create words out of two sounds (i.e., "ta" and "ble"). However, her ability to identify the sounds within words (her phonological awareness) was variable. Specifically, she could not identify common phonemes such as "p" and "b." When presented with visual cues, Sally was able to identify a pictured word that contained a given sound. However, on the WIAT-III she had difficulty independently identifying initial and ending sounds of words. For example, she reversed "bat" and "cat."

Sally was able to read several written words, including "they," "when," and "shop." Additionally, she was able to identify pictures matching up to two words, such as "two fish" and "red box." However, Sally struggled to sound out nonsense words. When letters were put into novel combinations, she was largely unable to identify and combine the correct letter sounds. For example, she said "rox" and "bix" when shown the nonsense word "rix." This performance reflects Sally's visual discrimination difficulties, as well as her variable understanding of letter-sound correspondence.

In terms of written work, Sally was able to clearly and correctly write an Average number of letters within a 30-second time limit. Notably, when asked to write the full alphabet, she revered the letters "j" and "z," and omitted the letter "n," again reflecting the effects of her visual discrimination and sequencing problems. She was able to write her name and the words "cat" and "in." However, she was inconsistent in her ability to write letters corresponding to sounds; while she correctly identified "a," "z," and "k," she wrote "g" as the letter corresponding with the "j" sound in "jump." She also wrote "dE (with the letter E backwards) for "be." This performance reflects Sally's inconsistent understanding of letter-sound correspondence as well as her visual discrimination and organization issues and tendency for letter reversal.

In sum, Sally's academic abilities were variable and compromised by her neurocognitive weaknesses. Specifically, her visual discrimination and organization difficulties compromised her ability to consistently identify abstract visual stimuli, such as letters and math symbols. Further, Sally's phonological awareness and understanding of letter-sound correspondence was variable and required remediation. Academic intervention was recommended, specifically, placement in a small, structured classroom geared to students with dyslexia.

Nonverbal Learning Disorder

Individuals with nonverbal learning disorders present with stronger language-based skills and weaker visual-spatial skills. This discrepancy is present in IQ tests, memory tasks and specific visual tests. Typically, these patients will also demonstrate poor math skills as well as poor organization, particularly with visual material (Thompson, 1997).

In the following case example, I present test findings from a patient with a nonverbal learning disorder. I am only including those sections that highlight her visual delays. This excerpt captures the significant impact of Nonverbal learning Disorder on developing visual skills. Her disabilities met criteria for academic accommodations, including extra time and academic support. (See Table 2.3.)

Charlotte was an 18-year-old young adult who was referred for a reassessment to get an updated picture of her functioning. Charlotte was diagnosed with Nonverbal Learning Disorder at a young age and has previously received intervention and academic accommodations.

Charlotte's cognitive abilities were assessed with the WAIS-IV, an individually administered test of intellectual strengths and weaknesses in both verbal and nonverbal domains. Charlotte obtained a Full Scale IQ of 95, indicating that her cognitive abilities are classified as Average compared to her

Table 2.3. Wechsler Adult Intelligence Scale—Fourth Edition: Charlotte

Scale/Subtest	*Index*	*Percentile*	*Qualitative Rating*
Full Scale IQ	**95**	**37th**	**Average**
Verbal Comprehension Index	**114**	**82nd**	**High Average**
Perceptual Reasoning Index	**84**	**14th**	**Low Average**
Working Memory Index	**111**	**77th**	**High Average**
Processing Speed Index	**71**	**3rd**	**Borderline**

Verbal Comprehension	**SS***		
Similarities	**10**		
Vocabulary	13		
Information	15		
Working Memory	**SS***		
Digit Span	15		
Arithmetic	9		
Perceptual Reasoning	**SS***		
Block Design	7		
Matrix Reasoning	6		
Visual Puzzles	9		
Processing Speed	**SS***		
Symbol Search	6		
Coding	3		

* >16 = Very Superior; 15–14 = Superior; 13–12 = High Average; 11–8 = Average; 7 = Low Average; <7 = Below Average

age peers. However, this score is likely an underestimate of her true cognitive potential due to her variable performance across and within tasks. Charlotte's Verbal Comprehension Index of 114 (82nd percentile) fell within the High Average range, as did her Working Memory Index of 111 (77th percentile). Charlotte's Perceptual Reasoning Index of 84 (14th percentile) fell within the Low Average range, while her Processing Speed Index of 71 (3rd percentile) fell within the Borderline range. The difference between Charlotte's visual and verbal abilities is considered statistically significant and reflects her nonverbal learning disability. An analysis of Charlotte's performance revealed considerable difficulties with visual organization, sequencing and discrimination, as well as exceptionally slow graphomotor speed. Areas of cognitive strength included a well-developed vocabulary and an excellent fund of general information, reflecting a strong ability to learn and recall verbal information and indicating strong academic potential.

Within the verbal domain, Charlotte demonstrated a sophisticated ability to understand verbal information and provide appropriate verbal responses. She demonstrated a very strong fund of general information, performing in the Superior range when asked questions including, "Who wrote Alice in Wonderland?" and, "Who was Catherine the Great?" Her word knowledge was also strong, and she scored within the High Average range when defining words, including "tirade" and "encumber."

Charlotte's perceptual reasoning skills, which include her nonverbal reasoning and perceptual organization abilities, were relatively weak and fell within the Low Average range. Her abstract visual problem solving, and visual sequencing abilities fell within the Below Average range when asked to analyze and complete visual patterns based on color, form and distribution in space (Matrix Reasoning). This was not due to her conceptual skills but rather reflects her slowed speed when it comes to visual processing and visual efficiency. Charlotte demonstrated poor visual-spatial reasoning and visual organization and planning abilities when asked to recreate graphic designs using colored blocks (Block Design).

Charlotte's working memory abilities, which refer to her capacity to store and manipulate verbal information in short term memory, were variable and ranged from Average to High Average. In general, her short-term memory for non-complex material is very strong. She was able to remember and recite strings of numbers verbatim and in reverse order; she had somewhat more difficulty after arranging the strings of numbers into numerical order, reflecting her difficulties with sequencing and organization typical of individuals with nonverbal learning disorder. Although in the Average range, her ability to mentally solve arithmetic word problems was significantly lower. Charlotte needed to have many of the items repeated and solved several outside of testing time limits.

Processing speed refers to the rate at which an individual processes simple or routine information. Charlotte's performance fell well below expected levels for her age and reflects an area of significant neurocognitive weakness. Her decision speed is very slow, and her visual discrimination and scanning skills are poor due to her nonverbal learning disorder. Thus, Charlotte will need more time than would be expected to complete most tasks involving visual information.

In sum, Charlotte had a well-developed vocabulary and a sophisticated fund of general knowledge, reflecting an excellent ability to learn and recall verbal information. Although Charlotte's performance on the WAIS-IV fell within the Average Range, her verbal skills were stronger than her other cognitive abilities. The difference between Charlotte's visual and verbal abilities was considered statistically significant and reflected her nonverbal learning disability. An analysis of Charlotte's performance revealed considerable difficulties with visual organization, sequencing and discrimination, as well as exceptionally slow decision making and graphomotor speed.

Attention Deficit Disorder

Individuals with attention deficit disorder present with significant impairment on tests of attention. In addition, on the WAIS or WISC IQ tests, scores on the Working Memory Index as well as the Processing Speed Index tend to be depressed. There may be an overall erratic quality to the academic and memory scores, reflecting inconsistent attention. Here is an excerpt of a report on an adolescent with attention deficit disorder.

Alex is a 12-year-old boy who was referred by his mother due to concerns regarding erratic academic performance. Alex was described as a bright youngster whose grades were inconsistent. The CPT was administered and confirmed the presence of attention difficulties (see Table 2.4). In addition, the SCAN-A Test of Auditory Processing indicated distractibility to noise, further confirming attentional issues. (See Table 2.5.)

Table 2.4. Conners Continuous Performance Test—Third Edition (CPT-3): Alex

Measure	*T-Score*	*Guideline*	*Interpretive Description*
Response Type			
Detectability (d′)	50	Average	Average ability to differentiate targets from non-targets
Error Type			
Omissions	47	Average	Average rate of missed targets
Commissions	32	Average	Average rate of incorrect responses to non-targets
Perseverations	64	Elevated	High rate of random, repetitive, or anticipatory responses
Reaction Time Statistics			
Hit Reaction Time (HRT)	54	Average	Average mean response speed
HRT Standard Deviation	66	Elevated	High inconsistency in reaction times
Variability	59	High Average	Slightly above average variability in reaction time consistency
HRT Block Change	52	Average	Average change in response speed in later blocks
HRT Inter-Stimulus Interval (ISI) Change	65	Elevated	Substantial reduction in response speed at longer ISIs

Table 2.5. A Test for Auditory Processing Disorder in Adolescents and Adults (SCAN-A): Alex

Subtest	*SS*	*PR*	*Qualitative*
Filtered Words	11	63	Average
Auditory-Figure Ground	6	9	Low
Competing Words	10	50	Average
Competing Sentences	12	75	High Average

Attention involves the ability to stay attuned to incoming stimuli or focus on a particular task while blocking out competing information. It also requires the ability to respond appropriately to stimuli, in other words, to either inhibit inappropriate responses or sustain appropriate responses without fatiguing. For optimal functioning, it is essential that an individual can sustain these abilities over time, particularly in academic settings. Alex's attentional abilities were measured by the Connors' Continuous Performance Test, Third Edition (CPT-III), the SCAN A, a test of auditory processing and attention, the Behavioral Assessment for Children, Third Edition (BASC-3), a questionnaire completed by both his mother and him, and behavioral observations made during the testing process.

The CPT-III required Alex to respond to stimuli on a computer, specifically to click the mouse or spacebar when a letter was present. It also asked him not to respond to similar but extraneous stimuli, thus requiring him to inhibit a response. This is a relatively dull test and requires fourteen minutes of sustained attention on a low-demand task. Because of its unchallenging nature, sustained attention to this task can be difficult. Alex's performance on the CPT-III showed indications of inattentiveness, difficulties with sustained attention, and difficulties with vigilance.

Alex's performance on the CPT-III also showed weaknesses in skills related to switching and sustaining attention over long periods of time. Alex had a high rate of perseverations, or random, repetitive, and anticipatory responses. This indicates that he had difficulty changing his pace regardless of the tempo of the task. This also shows that he had difficulty maintaining attention, which was also evident in several other areas. He showed high inconsistency in reaction time (HRT Standard Deviation), indicating variable attention to the task at hand. He also showed slower response speeds when the time between the stimuli was increased, suggesting that he experienced difficulties paying attention when he is bored or not constantly stimulated (HRT ISI Change).

While Alex's performance on the CPT-III shows difficulties in sustained attention to a relatively boring task, his difficulties with attention are not as evident elsewhere. On both his own and his mother's reports on the BASC-3, he fell in the normal range for attentional abilities. However, his mother reports that he sometimes struggles with organization and deadlines and is easily distracted. In contrast, when attending to social stimuli, such as listening to others speak and following directions, she reports he does well. On his own self-report questionnaire, Alex reports that, although he is forgetful and struggles to pay attention in school at times, he does not feel that he has a short attention span and does not receive such feedback from others. Alex demonstrated good attention throughout both testing sessions. While he became restless at times and asked how much longer the testing would take, he did not seem to waver or fatigue in his attentional abilities. The testing setting, however, is unique and different from other academic settings, where there are numerous students and instructors that are distracting. In sum, Alex's demonstrated attentional weaknesses on the CPT combined with his inconsistent processing speed indicate moderate difficulties with attention.

Alex's ability to process auditory stimuli was assessed with the SCAN-A. The SCAN-A consists of four subtests which tap auditory perceptual skills beyond the peripheral hearing mechanism. More specifically, the SCAN-A tests the ability to discriminate between background and foreground noise, attend to auditory stimuli, and discriminate between sound heard by the right and left ears. The subject is presented with distorted words and sentences that are conveyed via headphones and the subject is asked to guess the words that are mumbled or presented with background noise, which makes them difficult for people with auditory processing deficits to hear.

Alex's performance on this task revealed solid auditory attention and processing abilities, with one exception that fell into the Low Range. His scores were predominantly in the normal range, and he performed particularly well when asked to decipher sentences presented simultaneously in both ears (Competing Sentences, Scaled Score = 12, 75th percentile) and when asked to identify words that were muffled (Filtered Words, Scaled Score = 11, 63rd percentile). When asked to decipher words presented simultaneously in both ears, he performed in the Average Range (Competing Words, Scaled Score = 10, 50th percentile). He had the most trouble when asked to identify words presented in the presence of background noise (Auditory Figure Ground, Scaled Score = 6, 9th percentile, Low). This indicates that Alex is susceptible to being highly distracted and may struggle to hear instructions when there is a significant amount of background noise, which is very common in the classroom setting. This would thus impact his attentional abilities in school when listening to instruction and completing in-class assignments or tests. Alex would therefore benefit from working in more quiet spaces with less extraneous stimuli.

This report illustrates the complexity of attentional difficulties and the importance of a nuanced approach when diagnosing ADD.

High Functioning Autism

Individuals with high-functioning autism manifest inconsistencies throughout the testing. They are often highly verbal and academically skilled but display concrete thinking, social awkwardness, and erratic attention. Theory of Mind

Tests are crucial to understand the impact of this disorder as they evaluate the capability of the individual to consider someone else's perspective. Tests that assess understanding and recognition of emotions are also important components of the assessment. I will now present an excerpt of a report of a young man with autism.

Eugene is a 22-year-old young adult who was referred for testing to assess current level of functioning and to clarify diagnosis. Eugene has a long history of psychiatric and academic difficulties beginning in eighth grade where he demonstrated significant anxiety and depression. Currently, he is graduating from a private, special education program and planning to enroll in college. He is self-diagnosed with autism spectrum disorder. His scores on the Social Responsiveness Scale reflect the impact of his autism on social cognition, communication and motivation. (See Table 2.6.)

Information regarding Eugene's social, emotional, and behavioral functioning was gathered through projective measures, questionnaires, background information, and behavioral observations made during testing. Clinical impressions suggest that Eugene was pleasant, bright, and cooperative. There was no evidence of perceptual disturbance.

Eugene's parents described him as empathic and willing to go the "extra mile" for those who are in trouble. Eugene's responses on the Rorschach Inkblot Test, a projective measure that asks the individual what a blot "might be," indicated that Eugene was capable of thinking logically and coherently.

However, despite these strengths, Eugene struggled in a number of areas. He was highly anxious in the testing session and carries previous diagnoses of generalized and social anxiety disorder. Their father's responses on the BASC-3 placed Eugene's Anxiety scale in the Clinically Significant range. He indicated that Eugene was almost always fearful and nervous and almost always worries in general but also about things that cannot change and about making mistakes. Additionally, Eugene exhibited signs of depression, including suicidal thoughts. On the BASC-3, Mr. K indicated that Eugene was often sad, almost always seemed lonely, was easily upset, and cried easily.

Table 2.6. Social Responsiveness Scale—Second Edition (SRS-2): Eugene

Scale	*T-Score*	*Qualitative Rating*
Social Awareness	65	Moderate
Social Cognition	65	Moderate
Social Communication	57	Within Normal Range
Social Motivation	88	Severe
Repetitive Behavior	88	Severe
Total Score	**64**	**Mild**

Furthermore, Eugene exhibited many social difficulties and had trouble maintaining friendships during the COVID pandemic. Additionally, Eugene reported that he has trouble reading the non-verbal cues of others and interpreting facial expressions. Eugene also indicated that he copies others in social situations because he does not intuitively know how to behave or respond socially.

Eugene's parents each completed the Social Responsiveness Scale, Second Edition (SRS-2), a diagnostic questionnaire that identifies social impairment associated with autism spectrum disorder. Though they differed somewhat in their appraisal of their child's social responsiveness, they each identified Eugene's Social Motivation and Restricted Interests and Repetitive Behavior scales as areas of particular concern. Their responses indicated that Eugene never seems to mind being out of step with or not on the same wavelength as others, would almost always rather be alone than with others, almost always seems more fidgety in social situations than when alone, and is almost always too tense in social situations.

Eugene's responses on projective tests evidenced similar weaknesses. Results of the Rorschach Inkblot Test indicated that Eugene has limited capacity to form close attachments to other people and that they are less capable than their peers in navigating interpersonal situations. Similarly, his responses on the Thematic Apperception Test (TAT), a projective task on which he was asked to tell a story in response to ambiguous visual cues, were notable because he reported drawing upon movies and television shows to craft each story rather than creating his own original narratives, demonstrating difficulty with imagination, a characteristic feature of autism spectrum disorder.

Overall, Eugene is struggling with anxiety, low mood, and difficulty with social relatedness. It is likely that his low mood is related to their social challenges. As such, he would benefit from continued therapy, regular consultation with their psychiatrist, and continued development of coping strategies to help them navigate the social environment of college and beyond.

As can be seen from the above report, diagnosing high-functioning autism is complicated and requires attention to multiple factors including self-report, family observations, and performance on tests.

DEFICITS ARE RELATIVE

Diagnosis is an important part of the testing process, as can be seen from the above case examples. However, what is equally as important is a detailed and sophisticated analysis that compares the individual with his or her peers as well as the identification of unique strengths and weaknesses within the individual's learning profile. When evaluating deficits, it is important to keep in mind that deficits are relative to the individual and the goal of the neuropsychological evaluation is to create a comprehensive picture of the individual's neurocognitive strengths and weaknesses relative to him or herself.

Likewise, it is important to note that having a learning disorder does not mean that the individual is not intelligent. Some children and adults with LDs demonstrate superior IQ scores alongside significant neurocognitive challenges. These individuals have been termed "twice exceptional" insofar as they are both intellectually gifted and learning disabled. When evaluating those individuals with superior intellect, an Average score indicates an area of significant challenge. If an individual with Superior intelligence scores within the Average range on any task, this is considered an area of relative weakness and meets criteria for an LD.

Likewise, if the performance falls within the same range as other scores and is comparable to the individual's peers within a particular subgroup (see cultural issues below), then average or low average performance would not be indicative of a select neurocognitive deficit. In sum, it is crucial to consider the scores within the relevant context for the individual being evaluated.

NEUROPSYCHOLOGICAL FEEDBACK

Feedback is always given once the individual completes the test battery. The scores are reviewed with the patient and often the family as well as the school, therapist, tutor, and other allied professionals. Recommendations for services, school placement, and accommodations are discussed. Feedback can be a transformative experience for the individual and his or her family in terms of understanding diagnosis, gaining awareness of strengths and challenges, and benefitting from specific recommendations. It can also be a difficult experience for patients and families, who might find the diagnosis of a learning disability emotionally distressing.

Neuropsychological assessments are used to diagnose learning, attention, and psychiatric disorders, and to provide recommendations for how best to intervene when children present with these difficulties. Though procedural in nature, this process is often anything but academic. It can be intensely anxiety producing, stressful, and even shaming, and can leave both parents and their child feeling acutely exposed. The challenge, then, is to develop methods of engaging parents in a collaborative investigation into their child's struggles that avoids alienating or rigidifying their perspective. Rather than viewing testing as something that is done to the child, my goal is to find ways to reduce any asymmetry between tester and parent. Engaging parents as collaborators is the underlying principle guiding the concrete suggestions to follow.

It is equally important to create a collaborative relationship between child and tester. I will now discuss the therapeutic benefits and risks of feedback.

Although 71 percent of neuropsychologists in clinical practice conduct testing feedback sessions with patients (Pegg et al., 2008), best practices for providing assessment feedback to children and their families have received short shrift in the existing literature (Jacobson et al., 2015; Tharinger et al., 2008). Despite its popularity and perceived value (Meyer et al., 2001), the assessment process can be a source of significant frustration and anxiety for families (Westervelt et al., 2007). One common finding is that neuropsychological results are often poorly communicated by professionals and, consequently, misunderstood by parents and children (Donofrio et al., 1999). In the absence of widely understood best practices, we run the risk of leaving parents and children solely with negative feelings about themselves and their diagnoses.

Although most of the literature is focused on children, testing and feedback pose similar problems for adults. Adults come for assessment for a variety of reasons including concern about daily functioning, diagnosis, recommendations for medication and intervention. The same techniques we are discussing for children apply for adults.

In successful feedback sessions, the clinician adequately explains how psychological and neurological factors contribute to a child's academic, social, and emotional difficulties. This information is intended to guide patients and families in pursuing treatment and accessing academic resources. I will hereafter discuss methods for avoiding common pitfalls while ensuring that the test results will be positively received by parents and children.

I vividly recall a formative experience I had with a patient's father over twenty-five years ago, when I was just beginning my career as a neuropsychologist. My comprehensive assessment of his son led me to diagnose him with attention deficit disorder (ADD). My perspective on this diagnosis was positive; the son could now receive treatment and in-school accommodations to enhance his academic success. However, during the feedback session, the father became increasingly agitated and insisted that his son did not have ADD. I found myself embroiled in a power struggle with the father that resulted in him angrily leaving my office.

I later realized that I had neglected and misinterpreted the father's considerable anxiety surrounding his son's deficits. Because I insisted on a strong diagnosis without attending to the father's anxiety, a good testing experience resulted in a bad clinical outcome. This experience, (among others) motivated me to devise a better code of conduct for my feedback sessions that aims to lessen stress and enhance collaboration between myself and the families and children I treat.

Feedback may have therapeutic effects on both parents and their children (Finn and Tonsager, 1997; Gorske, 2008; Hamilton et al., 2009). Human and Teglasi (1993) reported favorable changes in parents' self-reports following feedback, including improved parent-child relationships. How might testers leverage the positive effects of feedback? The information testers need to impart exposes the child's difficulties and elicits diverse responses. The parents' anxiety about their child's future is often triggered; their wishes for their child may make it difficult to hear the feedback. However, parents who are encouraged to voice their concerns often come away with a better understanding of their children's challenges. Further, explaining the nature of the deficit by using specific examples that relate directly to the patient's and family's concerns can greatly facilitate insight into the disorder and receptiveness to intervention. A clinical example illustrates this principle:

> An eleventh grader, Sarah, was referred to me due to concern about performance anxiety about her schoolwork, which manifested in her avoiding her work, "spacing out," and becoming easily frustrated. The evaluation revealed significant attentional deficits. Feedback with the parents focused on explaining that she has difficulty focusing, sitting and focusing on her work, and completing tasks in an efficient manner. Sarah confirmed that she is easily distracted and procrastinates. As the parents understood that they had misinterpreted her attentional deficits as anxiety, their concerns were reassured, and they arranged to consult with a psychopharmacologist for medicine for Sarah. Understanding the specific symptoms of ADD that Sarah was displaying at home, that is, procrastinating and not doing her work paved the way to effective intervention.

What should a tester do when parents seem reluctant to abandon the notion that their child is lazy, stupid, or otherwise defective? It can be frustrating and upsetting for the tester when parents continue to blame their child and/or reject useful feedback. In these cases, it is helpful for the tester to take a long-term view. It is important to remember that the process can demand an incubation period during which the family digests this information. This can help counter parents' resistance and give them room to assimilate test results gradually. Allowing the parents to fully voice their concerns can also diminish resistance to testing feedback. When this approach is not sufficient, I refer to an outside therapist to work through the family's entrenched ideas.

I recently consulted with a bright 19-year-old who had failed his first semester of college. His driven, high-achieving mother readily acknowledged that her son was diagnosed with ADHD at age seven and required extensive intervention throughout his compulsory education. Still, she expressed frustration with her son and described him as "parasitic and lazy." She expressed bewilderment with regard to her son's lack of motivation and contrasted her own work ethic with his difficulties. By leveraging the test results, empathizing with the mother's feelings, and engaging in parent guidance sessions over a six-month period, we were able to achieve an improved parent-child relationship. In this case, the key to treatment was focusing on increasing the mother's understanding of the severity of her son's attention and learning difficulties. Patiently educating her on the neurocognitive challenges her son faced helped her eventually reframe his issues; together, they were then able to devise realistic educational and professional plans he successfully implemented.

CONCLUSION

Evaluating children, adolescents, and adults with neurocognitive impairments is the first step to establishing a diagnosis, creating a comprehensive learning profile, and providing a road map for treatment and intervention. There is a plethora of assessment instruments that can be used, the detailed discussion of which is beyond the scope of this book. However, familiarity with a core battery and having some ability to interpret the results is helpful for successful psychotherapy with patients with neurocognitive challenges. To give a fuller picture of a neuropsychological evaluation, I present a complete test report in the appendix.

CONCLUSION

Chapter Three

The Emotional Impact of Neurocognitive Challenges

It is well understood that neurocognitive challenges negatively impact one's ability to function, both academically and professionally. The connection between learning and attention disorders and poor performance in school and on the job is straightforward. For example, a struggling reader is diagnosed with dyslexia and recommended for specific interventions to support reading skills. However, the social and emotional sequelae of learning and attention disorders are often neglected—although they are critical to understand if these patients are to receive therapeutic help. To enter into the psyche of an individual with neurocognitive impairment, it is crucial to understand how his or her specific deficits impact his or her self-esteem, emotional regulation skills, interpersonal relationships, and overall mental health (Johnson, 2005).

Psychiatric disorders are two-to-four times as common in children with learning disabilities compared to those without, with an estimated 30–50 percent of such children having a mental disorder in a study using the DSM-IV for diagnosis (Dekker & Koot, 2003). Similarly, Sahoo et al. (2015), in a population-based survey, documented that about 30 percent of children with specific learning disabilities in India also demonstrated significant emotional and behavioral problems, such as depression, anxiety, suicidal ideation, and substance abuse. In findings from the National Longitudinal Study of Adolescent Health, adolescents with learning disabilities had twice the risk of emotional distress as compared with neurotypical peers and females with learning disorders were at twice the risk of attempting suicide compared to their peers (Svetaz et al., 2001). In addition, a survey study by Johnson (2005) indicates that painful feelings, such as shame and guilt, are prevalent among individuals with neurocognitive challenges, contributing to psychosocial difficulties. Extensive case histories with theoretical underpinnings have similarly documented an elevated incidence of psychiatric issues and emotional distress among individuals with neurocognitive challenges (Orenstein, 2000; Conway, 2017; Cohen, 1987).

Gardner (1980) provides an evocative description of treatment with adults with Minimal Brain Dysfunction (the older term for learning and attention deficits). He astutely notes that the therapist can be most helpful by appreciating how "the neurological deficits interfere with his or her social functioning." He delineates the toll on self-esteem and relationships due to impulsivity and distractibility. He further outlines how self-worth is negatively affected by disparaging evaluations of the patient by parents and teachers. Thus, the interaction between learning disabilities and mental health is crucial and clearly needs to be addressed.

SELF-ESTEEM

Having a learning disability significantly impacts a child's ability to develop a positive sense of self and leads to disturbances in self-esteem, mood regulation, and interpersonal relationships. Children may suffer from the experience of failing to live up to their own standards, as well as to those of parents, teachers and peers. Palombo (2001) notes that intelligent children with learning disabilities often feel intense shame, primarily due to their struggles achieving academic goals. They realize that, although they are smart, they cannot demonstrate their full competence. I have noticed how this experience of frequently missing the mark in school compromises one's ability to develop a unified and positive sense of self, and to progress socially as well as academically.

Osman (2000) noted that youngsters with learning disabilities tend to have low self-esteem and negative attributions for success. They are more likely to attribute success or failure to external circumstances, such as "luck." In addition, the lower their self-esteem, the more likely they are to attribute their failures to being incompetent (Grolnick & Ryan, 1990).

After repeated failures, children develop learned helplessness, a term coined by Seligman (1975). They believe they are incapable of succeeding; thus, they do not exert effort and then fall further behind their peers, academically and socially. The following case example illustrates this pattern.

Charlotte, a bright young adult, was completing a graduate program in history at a prestigious college. Previously diagnosed with a Nonverbal Learning Disability (as described in Chapter 2), she had difficulty with organization, time management, and completing reading and writing tasks efficiently. She worked slowly despite a good grasp of the material. Her struggles to complete her thesis were marked by procrastination and difficulty submitting her work on time. She admitted that she was adopting a "blasé attitude" because she was scared she would become overwhelmed with anxiety and depression and then not be able to complete any work. She expressed her frustration that she could not keep up with her peers and poignantly described her desire to be "normal." She described being pulled out of class when she was younger and getting teased by her peers. She was reluctant to ask for help for fear of being judged negatively and rejected even by tutors and learning specialists. As such, she set up a vicious cycle where herself criticism led to avoidance, which interfered with her ability to complete her work, which in turn only fueled her self-criticism.

The humiliation suffered by students with learning disabilities is multifaceted. For one, repeated experiences of difficulty with mastering information and skills lead to shame and frustration. Additionally, most children are acutely aware of the social hierarchy and pecking order. When they are singled out for special instruction or services, it is highly stigmatizing, both due to their own self-consciousness and because of others' reactions and comments. Consequently, children will often avoid subjects they have difficulty with by claiming they do not like them, or that they are "bad" at them—which robs them of the opportunity for mastery, further compromising their self-esteem. The following case example illustrates this defense mechanism.

Adam, an engaging twelfth grader, was referred for testing after failing several courses at his school. He expressed that he was "unmotivated" and thus did not complete any assignments. This pattern of avoidance of work had been established for many years despite his parents "yelling" at him and his own awareness that he needed to complete his work. He was convinced that he simply did not want to do the work. Testing revealed significantly slowed speed, attention deficits and poor organization. When I explained to Adam that his lack of "motivation" was due to neurocognitive challenges that made reading and writing slow, laborious, and frustrating, he responded that it "made sense" to him although he continued to express the idea that he was "unmotivated," that is, the issue was volitional. I explained that he lacked sufficient support and accommodations to help him with his work despite an excellent conceptual grasp of the material. With academic support and extended time in place, Adam began to complete his work and was then able to express pride in his accomplishments.

Although patients feel intense shame regarding their challenges, they may not be able to label or identify their challenges accurately. Frequently, the patients view the learning disorder as all-encompassing and feel defined by their condition. They perceive themselves as globally inadequate, as "bad," "lazy," and "stupid." They do not understand that their difficulties are limited to specific cognitive functions and do not reflect their global intelligence, motivation, or aptitude.

A crucial principle in therapy is to understand that learning disorders are neurocognitive and need to be treated as a biological condition that the person must recognize and to which they must adapt. Gensler (1993) suggests that clinicians treat these defects as a "given[,] and to address their elaboration in character, defense and relational style." His perspective is that the therapist must understand the neurocognitive challenges as part of the patients' "hard wiring" and should be treated as part of the patient's biological makeup. The focus should be on how the patient can adapt to their challenges and compensate successfully.

THE MYTH OF LAZINESS

The myth of laziness is a particularly potent example of self-blame when presented with neurocognitive impairment. I frequently hear either a teacher or parent describe the child as lazy, or sometimes the patient will describe themselves as such. It is a dismissive, catch-all phrase that serves to mask the underlying issues and further contributes to the problem. A case example will illustrate the toxic impact of this issue.

> Matthew, a highly intelligent, personable teenager was referred for therapy due to depression. He described feeling "lazy," and socially withdrawn. For example, he preferred to stay in his room rather than eat dinner with his family, had difficulty reaching out to friends, and would procrastinate on assignments. Testing revealed significant attention and auditory processing deficits. Once Matthew understood that his withdrawal and preference to be in his room was related to both organizational difficulties and noise sensitivity, he was able to strategize on how to effectively socialize and complete his work. Although the idea of his "laziness" still came up in therapy periodically, he was able to be more effective academically and socially.

Many of my patients poignantly recall the angry and frustrated responses to their struggles with learning and comprehension. They tell of parents, teachers, and tutors asking, "How could you not know this? I already explained it to you ten times!" This type of treatment leads a child with learning disabilities to blame themselves for their difficulties, internalizing a self-image of someone who is "stupid, lazy, or both" (Kelly & Ramundo, 2006).

INTERPERSONAL RELATIONSHIPS

There is extensive literature documenting the social challenges of children with learning disabilities (Bender and Wall, 1994; Osman, 1995). Youngsters with learning disabilities often have difficulty understanding emotional and social situations (Bryan, 1991; Osman, 1995). Likewise, deficits in socially acceptable behaviors and acceptance by peers have been described in children and adolescents with learning disabilities (Vaughn & LaGreca, 1993). This leads us to ask, what are some of the underlying reasons behind this significant problem?

Children with learning disorders are frequently misunderstood, as they have difficulty communicating, which may lead to impaired interpersonal relationships with peers and adults. For example, in a study using the Profile of Nonverbal Sensitivity (PONS), adolescents with poor auditory, visual, and multi-sensory perception skills had significant difficulty understanding nonverbal social information (Sisterhen & Gerber, 1989).

As an indirect consequence of their learning deficits, neurodivergent children receive more than their fair share of parents and teachers expressing disappointment in them and even rejecting them based on both their academic and social performance. As individuals with learning disorders are vulnerable to these types of rejection, they may then avoid academic or social situations that pose the risk of similarly painful experiences. The awareness that they are "different" from their peers and are falling short of expectations often leads to an anxious/avoidant attachment style. Children will often make statements such as "nobody likes me," and " the teacher hates me"—which are merely expressions of frustration with their compromised social relationships. In addition, children with neurocognitive challenges are frequent targets of bullying, as bullies can sense and then target their feelings of low self-esteem. Further, they often lack the social skills to successfully advocate for themselves and thus prevent the bullying. Clinically, my neurodivergent patients uniformly report having experienced severe bullying which has left significant emotional scars and led to profound social anxiety and isolation. In fact, Fogler et al. (2020) propose that bullying is directly associated with having ADHD. A recent survey in Greece showed that 40 percent of students with learning disabilities suffer from bullying at school (Panastasiou, 2018). The following case example illustrates this negative cycle.

During a group therapy session with young adults with neurocognitive challenges, the topic of bullying came up; the group members shared their experiences of being bullied by peers in elementary school. They discussed not being able to engage in the quick childhood banter of the playground and thus subsequently becoming the target of mean comments, exclusion from games, and even physical violence. These experiences then translated into avoidance of social situations as teenagers and adults due to anxiety about being rejected. Role playing in the group and experience of the group as a successful social outlet facilitated improved interpersonal skills.

Lastly, children with learning disorders, attention deficit disorders, and high-functioning autism demonstrate a higher incidence of parent-child conflict and impaired family relationships (Sundheim & Voeler, 2004). In fact, parent-child conflict is an early sign of potential language difficulty (Cohen et al., 1999; Jenkins et al., 1980). Parents often misunderstand their child's behavior and misattribute their lack of compliance with rules and expectations (Cohen et al., 1993). For example, children are seen as "oppositional" or "stubborn" when they do not understand what is being asked of them. Sadly, these mismatches in communication can lead to the child's development of insecure attachment as the parents become dismissive and withdrawn due to their frustration with the child's behavior or learning difficulties (Capoizzi et al., 2007).

IDENTITY DEVELOPMENT

Unsurprisingly, neurodivergent children also struggle with identity development, a central problem which may undergird many other problems. Kohut (1971) describes the process whereby children internalize positive self-images in response to succeeding at tasks and obtaining approval from parents and teachers. As life presents frustration and challenges, the child is able to persevere, accomplish tasks, take pride in his or her performance and learn from mistakes. It is the mastering of challenges that underlies stable self-confidence. Identifying with the parent or teacher who has already succeeded at these tasks gives children the support and confidence they need to triumph. Learning is an optimal environment for this process as it is strewn with minor obstacles to be overcome. However, children with neurocognitive impairment are faced with overwhelming challenges that they cannot conquer successfully, particularly in a learning environment. Thus, they develop a negative self-image, and this transfers to relationships with friends, family members, and teachers.

Neurodivergent children are not able to successfully attain the goals that are expected of them and that they see the adults in their lives have achieved, and as happens in typical development. Ordinarily, children look to the parent as a role model and establish their identity in accordance with what the parent espouses. However, if a child feels that he or she is constantly falling short of the parent's standards, the child will not feel capable or competent to identify with the parent and the parent's ideals, and thus will develop myriad coping defenses—including withdrawal from the challenging tasks (mainly academic), oppositional, feelings of defeat, denial of his or her failures, and/or denial of the desire to identify with the parent (Kohut & Strozier, 1985). This will often extend to therapy; the child may be extraordinarily defensive and guarded in therapy, particularly when they fear that their deficits might be exposed.

THE IMPOSTER SYNDROME

Even when deficits are not exposed, individuals with learning and attention deficits can feel insecure in their identity and social role. Frequently, children and adolescents with neurocognitive challenges experience an "imposter syndrome," that is, the feeling that they are "fakes" who are "fooling" adults and peers and will be found out for being incapable. Repeatedly guessing when presented with challenges and "winging it" on tasks engenders feelings of a false self (Winnicott, 1960). These patients are painfully aware of their deficits, and believe they are tricking those around them by hiding or covering up their difficulties. Reliance on tutors and academic support can convince young adults that they were cheating; even getting extended time on tests can feel like gaming the system. This case example illustrates this clinical issue.

> Scott, a bright, high-achieving young adult, reported feeling like a "fraud" because he had never completed one book despite his impressive academic success. He received his diagnosis of dyslexia with relief and shamefacedly confessed that he had lied throughout his career about reading as he found it impossible to get through books due to his slowed reading speed.

AFFECT REGULATION

Affect regulation is a critical skill that is integral to development and often an area of concern for children with neurocognitive challenges. Children and adults who are poorly regulated manifest a limited ability to cope with stress, compromised interpersonal relationships, and intrapsychic volatility that significantly impairs social and academic progress. Maladaptive emotional regulation in children with varied cognitive challenges has been linked to poor working memory, rigidity, and impulsivity (Parvinchi et al., 2021). Additionally, problems with executive function impair impulse control and hence affect regulation (Hallowell & Ratey, 1994).

Language development is intimately related to affect regulation as children learn how to "use their words" instead of acting out when frustrated or angry. If children do not have the words to mediate their feelings and to help them think through the situation before acting on it, they may react impulsively, and even aggressively. It can also be extremely frustrating for them if they cannot convey their thoughts and feelings with language. When they cannot properly express themselves, children often resort to temper tantrums and aggressive behaviors to communicate their needs and desires. These behaviors unsurprisingly elicit negative responses from others, further damaging their self-esteem and social confidence (Silver, 2006).

The "fight/flight/freeze" response to trauma can be used as a lens into the experience of a child with learning problems in school. This model by Walter Cannon is now widely popularized as a way of understanding and treating anxiety and stress (Greenberg, 2016). School-related tasks become anxiety triggers, leading to the response cycle described by Cannon. Children initially enter school looking forward to the social and academic experience. As it becomes clear to them that they are not able to operate on the same level as their peers, their coping responses become characterized by a traumatic cycle. They often attempt to avoid the academic tasks (flight), lash out at peers or teachers (fight), or completely shut down (freeze). These responses may accompany them throughout their academic career and may also transfer to social situations. As noted above, difficulty with academic tasks causes children to come up with their own ideas as to the origin of their deficits; for example, they see themselves as any combination of lazy, stupid, bad, a failure, and incompetent. These self-percepts, often reinforced by parents, teachers, and peers, have a toxic impact on self-esteem and confidence and, consequently, the ability to develop frustration tolerance and grit.

In sum, the socioemotional sequelae of learning and attention deficits include low self-esteem, compromised affect regulation, difficulty establishing a positive and stable identity and compromised interpersonal relationships. Each specific neurocognitive impairment has a unique profile allowing us to understand the child's struggles more in depth. Thus, I will now discuss each profile separately with the accompanying social/emotional implications.

LANGUAGE BASED LEARNING DISORDER

Patients with language-based learning disorders typically present with relatively weak language skills and stronger visual-spatial skills. These individuals may have difficulty with reading and writing, and typically perform better on subjects such as math and science. Patients with language-based learning disorders often complain of being "tongue tied," not being able to engage in banter, and having difficulty with comprehending directions and instructions as compared with their peers. As they often cannot initiate or sustain conversation, they are at a significant social disadvantage. These patients are often mislabeled as "oppositional" or "resistant" due to their compromised expressive language skills. Likewise, participating in class is an area of anxiety for them, and they are often criticized for their perceived unwillingness to participate (Sorscher, 2022). The high prevalence of emotional and behavioral problems among children with speech, language, and communication disorders has been documented in a survey study (Prizant et al., 1990).

These challenges have a profound impact on these patients' sense of competence in academic and social arenas. They may become exceptionally reserved and anxious in social situations, including with family members, and may have significant difficulty advocating for themselves. Developmentally, they may suffer as they shy away from growth-producing social situations and thus do not get the opportunity to practice social skills and hold their own with group banter. A case example illustrates the significant impact of a language-based learning disorder on social skills and the emergence of an anxious/avoidant approach to social situations.

> Michael, a 25-year-old graduate student, struggles with expressive language skills. During group therapy, he often becomes "tongue tied" and visibly struggles with expressing his thoughts, often exclaiming in frustration, "Words!" Although Michael is motivated to socialize, and has several close friends, he spends most of his time alone and isolated as he is reluctant to approach people and seek out social situations. Through his work in the group, he began reaching out more regularly to his friends and even put up an online dating profile. These forays were extensively discussed and role-played in the group to help him improve his social confidence and ability to articulate his thoughts.

NONVERBAL LEARNING DISORDER

In contrast to the language-based learning disorders, individuals with nonverbal learning disabilities often present with strong language skills and compromised visual-spatial skills. Consequently, they may struggle to understand the nonverbal nuances of interpersonal interaction and communication. In addition, they often present with time management issues, compromised organizational skills and "sloppy" habits—for example, their personal hygiene is often poor, and their rooms and workspaces are often untidy. These patients are often misperceived as "flighty" and "needy," as their deficits make it difficult to be reliable and complete tasks without support. These difficulties compromise their social functioning as their peers, teachers, and family members are put off by these behaviors (Sorscher, 2022; Thompson, 1997).

Socially, they may misperceive facial expressions and have difficulty "reading the room." They may not understand hierarchies, as understanding proximal relationships requires visual-spatial and organizational skills that are often compromised in this population. As such, the child is unaware of the "pecking order" and may inadvertently offend others as a result. Thus, they may address a teacher or parent as one would address a peer or tell an unintentionally offensive anecdote. This is the child who clumsily trips over peers in the playground, chimes in with a joke once everyone has stopped laughing and avoids eye contact. In a sense they are "tone deaf," meaning they do not perceive interpersonal nuances the way their neurotypical peers do, and thus they can be perceived as disrespectful, shy, aloof, or rude. Therefore, they may experience significant rejection from peers and adults, leading to a damaged sense of self and profound insecurity in social situations (Sorscher, 2022).

Charlotte, the young adult with NVLD from the previous chapter, demonstrates significant social anxiety and has experienced bullying and rejection due to her neurocognitive difficulties. In elementary school, she was the target of bullying as she did not understand how to conduct herself on the playground and tended to demonstrate poor hygiene with a runny nose and dirty hands. In addition, she was clumsy and could not engage in either banter or the playground games. In college, her roommate requested a transfer because she could not keep the room clean. These experiences of social rejection lead to intense emotional distress and social isolation. Currently, Charlotte has developed a good social network but continues to require support to connect with new peers and network in a professional setting.

Other specific learning disorders include dyscalculia (compromised math skills), dysgraphia (deficient graphomotor skills), and dyslexia (poor reading skills). These specific learning challenges are related to the broader categories of language-based and nonverbal learning disorders, but do not necessarily share all the features of the larger categories and typically do not meet full criteria for diagnosis of either disorder. These students demonstrate significantly impaired academic performance and require intense remediation as well as accommodations to help them succeed academically. Auditory Processing Disorder is another diagnosis, in which individuals have difficulty processing auditory information. The psychological sequelae for these challenges are similar to those for the learning disorders described above.

ATTENTION DEFICIT DISORDER

When people have inattentive ADD they are seen as "spacy" and dreamy, whereas those with the hyperactive type of ADD are impulsive with poor self-regulation. As the DSM-V TR has consolidated the diagnosis into ADHD, we will be referring to all types of attention disorders as ADHD with the understanding that the diagnosis is along a continuum and spans a spectrum of symptoms from motor restlessness to lack of focus. The psychological consequences for both of these disorders include low self-esteem, isolation, anxiety, and depression. Inattentiveness is marked by a quiet withdrawal from tasks, "spacing out," doodling, and daydreaming. Inattentive children often miss information and have difficulty performing as a result. They may receive negative feedback for their "dreaminess," both from peers and adults. Socially, they may have difficulty sustaining friendships and following conversations as they tend to lose focus, "zone out," and become distracted. Their distractibility and tendency to go off on tangents in conversation makes them appear to be unempathic and insensitive as friends.

Children with attention deficit disorder (ADHD) frequently exhibit impaired executive functioning along with inattentiveness and poor impulse control. In addition, their organizational difficulties strongly hamper their ability to navigate the logistics of social events, as they have trouble organizing and following through on plans. They may forget to show up at a mutually agreed upon time, inadvertently stranding a friend who will then be reluctant to reschedule. They are often late to events and have significant time management issues, causing their family, friends, teachers, and bosses to erroneously conclude that they "don't care" and are not prioritizing the event or task, or are not exerting sufficient effort. These messages are often internalized, and the person with ADHD may see themselves as "bad," "lazy," and "stupid." Another common reaction to attentional issues in the classroom is to become the "class clown" and disrupt the lesson due to poor impulse control, low frustration tolerance, and a desire for peer approval. Their impulsivity also hinders their ability to relate to peers, as they may blurt out something insulting or simply not have the attention span to listen to a long story.

For children with attention deficit disorder, the ability to create and sustain a solid and positive self-image is hampered by the erratic and inconsistent quality of their work, relationships, and affect regulation (McCarthy & Conway 2011). They cannot rely on themselves to fully deliver on their goals, so they end up in an untenable situation, either enduring the frustration and disappointment that comes from not being able to produce or withdrawing from the task by procrastinating and coming up with maladaptive strategies to get their work done—such as lying, cheating, and submitting assignments at the last minute. Sometimes they can complete their work as the deadline approaches, as the adrenaline kicks in and they are finally able to focus. Nonetheless, their work is still done in haste and often falls short of the requirements. This disastrous cycle can continue for many years and leads to significant dysfunction, particularly as children mature and need to expand their academic/professional goals. A case example will illustrate the significant impact of ADHD symptoms on self-esteem and the ability to integrate a positive self-concept.

Cara, a bubbly, outgoing high school student, was constantly "getting in trouble" at home, in school and socially due to disruptive behaviors. She frequently interrupted in class, was late to all social and academic obligations, disregarded rules and seemed to have a blasé attitude when confronted. She was bewildered by the negative attention she received and said "Nobody likes me, I'm not popular, and the teachers are out to get me." At home, there was intense conflict regarding her room and difficulty complying with expectations. Cara expressed frustration and confusion; she felt unlovable, and despaired that she would ever attain her goals of social and academic success. With medication, therapy, and parent counseling, Cara was able to manage her attentional symptoms. She stopped getting in trouble, formed a group of friends, and performed better academically. This in turn had a strong reparative effect on her self-esteem.

AUTISM SPECTRUM DISORDER (ASD)

Individuals with Autism Spectrum Disorder have profound social and emotional challenges. In fact, the primary deficit is affective and interpersonal as people with ASD do not process or express emotions the way their typically developing peers do. Communication is often impaired, and these individuals have difficulty comprehending metaphorical or ambiguous language (Goldstein et al., 1994). In addition, limited use of vocal inflection, eye contact and recognition of nonverbal cues negatively impact social skills. (Yirmiya and Sigman, 1991). These individuals often have blank expressions, respond oddly to either exciting or sad news, and have difficulty offering comfort or support. Sturrock et al. (2021) described the impact of subtle language and communication difficulties on the emotional well-being of children with autism. The children described impaired functioning in school, with family members, and socially due to poor communication skills, which in turn leads to anxiety and low self-esteem.

For example, Eugene, a young adult with ASD who identifies as nonbinary (referenced in Chapter 2) recounted that, as a young child, their peers, teachers, and parents often asked them if they were upset when they were not because their facial expression unwittingly communicated distress. They learned to "mask" or assume a "happy expression" at all times, which then became a source of frustration, as it was a significant strain to maintain an artificial smile.

Individuals with ASD often lack empathy or "theory of mind" and cannot put themselves in another person's shoes. Thus, they may not react at all when their friend is distressed. They are often sincere and caring people who genuinely care about their friends but cannot truly empathize due to their deficits in social cognition. Likewise, they are prone to expressing their concern in a stiff, awkward, or rigid manner. In addition, they may engage in off-putting, "matter-of-fact" statements that they see as reasonable but that come across as overly blunt and tactless, as they cannot gauge the impact of their comments on the other person. A case example can illustrate the impact of ASD on social skills.

Leslie, a 30-year-old young adult with ASD, expressed frustration regarding her interaction with a job counselor. She mentioned that the counselor was looking for her to express interest or enthusiasm about various job opportunities, but Leslie did not feel happy about any of the openings. She said that she wants to work and would be grateful for any job but knew that she was not capable of expressing joy. I communicated to the counselor that Leslie was a responsible, diligent, and committed worker who would be satisfied with a structured job but lacked the capacity to communicate any specific interests or enthusiasms.

These deficits can often render initiating and sustaining friendships very difficult for individuals with ASD. Although they desire friends, they often lack the skills and affective range to engage in social situations. They are often aware of their deficiencies, and this awareness can lead to intense anxiety, depression, and self-criticism. White et al. (2009) documented that anxiety is common in children and adolescents with autism spectrum disorders, thus requiring attention and intervention.

TWICE EXCEPTIONAL CHILDREN

Many gifted children are "double labeled"—that is, they are intellectually gifted and learning disabled and demonstrate emotional, social, and behavioral problems (David, 2017). These twice exceptional children require accommodations for their deficits as well as a rigorous curriculum to ensure that their intellect is stimulated in school. These children are at particular risk for being misunderstood and misdiagnosed, as parents, teachers, and peers may not understand the juxtaposition of their high intelligence with their learning struggles.

LONG-RANGE IMPLICATIONS

In many cases, children and adults can compensate so successfully for their areas of neurocognitive weakness that they may go undiagnosed for many years. Nevertheless, individuals with attention and learning disabilities can still suffer from profound functional and emotional challenges. Attention deficit hyperactivity disorder and autism spectrum disorder are early onset disorders that extend into adulthood and are associated with poor academic skills as well as language deficits in adult life (Riglin et al., 2020). What we call a learning disability in childhood often develops into difficulties with exercising higher cognitive capacities and problem-solving abilities in adulthood (Gensler, 1993). Bucholtz (1987) comments that patients with neurocognitive disabilities bring a childhood history of emotional suffering caused by a legacy of learning failures and humiliations. Thus, it is important to take a comprehensive social/emotional/health/educational history of the patient when starting therapy. This step is critical when treating adolescents and adults as learning and/or attention disorders can be hidden, compensated for and go undiagnosed but still have profound implications for the patient in every arena.

Particularly with bright and capable adults, learning and attention disorders often get overlooked in treatment, and neurocognitive symptoms are thought to have a psychiatric etiology. I often have occasion to test adults who have not been previously diagnosed and frequently uncover learning disorders that they compensated for in childhood—but were a source of shame and anxiety.

A very successful advertising executive came in for testing because he was having difficulty keeping up with the demands of his job. When asked about his history, he disclosed that he was an erratic student whose scores were variable and that he was often criticized for "lack of effort." He excelled at his previous job but began to have performance difficulties after the company was sold. Test results revealed that he had mild attention issues as well as visual processing deficits that contributed to slowed speed and significant time management issues. These deficits were hampering his performance in his new position, as all business was conducted via email. He missed the face-to-face contact and verbal interactions that helped structure his work and contributed to his effectiveness. If his therapist had only focused on his anxiety and depression, his neurocognitive issues would not have been uncovered and he would have missed out on being able to improve his work life and mental health by recognizing these issues and taking steps to compensate for them.

In conclusion, the social and emotional sequelae of neurocognitive challenges are profound and far reaching. Neurodivergence is associated with anxiety, depression, low self-esteem, and interpersonal difficulties. In order to help the individual successfully resolve his or her difficulties, it is critical to understand the specific contribution of learning and attention challenges on identity formation, interpersonal skills, and psychopathology. The following chapters will address intervention, both neurocognitively and psychiatrically, to benefit these patients.

Chapter Four

Accommodations, Modifications, and Common Emotional Responses to Assistive Methods

Once students have been assessed and their neurocognitive challenges identified, the intervention plan typically includes assistive methods, including academic accommodations and/or classroom modifications. Accommodations involve the alteration of environment, curriculum, and equipment. Since accommodations do not alter what is being taught, instructors should be able to implement the same grading scale for students with disabilities as they do for students without disabilities. Examples include extended time for students with learning disabilities and large print books and worksheets for students with visual impairments. Accommodations are considered "reasonable and appropriate" to the extent that they remove disability-related barriers so that students with disabilities are afforded the same access to learning and opportunity to demonstrate knowledge and skills as a non-disabled peer (Hatcher & Waguespack, 2004).

Modifications are made for students with disabilities who are unable to comprehend all the content an instructor is teaching. These involve a change in curriculum and classroom content to adapt to the students' needs. For example, assignments might be reduced in number and significantly simplified for an elementary school student with cognitive impairments that limit his or her ability to understand the content taught in a general education class.

This chapter will first explore the legal context for implementing these assistive methods. I will then outline the types of accommodations and modifications most commonly used and differentiate them according to the specific disorder. I will next discuss why these interventions are important and address evidence supporting their efficacy. Common emotional responses to accommodations will also be discussed, as well as typical misconceptions by students and faculty. Lastly, case studies will be presented with the lens on how therapists can help patients who need to use these resources.

LEGAL MANDATE

The push to provide public education for students with disabilities began with a series of court cases culminating in a federal law requiring that all schools who receive federal funds provide adequate education for students with disabilities (Yell et al., 2008). Throughout the United States, from preschool through high school, students who are assessed and identified with learning disabilities, attention deficits, or autism may receive an Individualized Education Plan (IEP) that outlines needed services (Florell & Strait, 2020). The IEP is an in-depth, comprehensive, and goal-oriented document that outlines strengths, challenges, goals, and measurement criteria for each academic or social/emotional sphere. Alternatively, students may qualify for a 504 accommodation, if they have a disability that significantly impacts them in either academic, physical, or social domains. This is a cursory one-page document that outlines the disability and delineates the specific recommendation (Martin & Zirkel, 2011).

On a college level, the Rehabilitation Act of 1973 and the Americans with Disabilities Act of 1990 mandate services for students with disabilities in order for them to receive equal access to education (McCusker, 1994). In addition, the No Child Left Behind Act of 2001 attempted to bring greater accountability nationwide by mandating the inclusion of all students in statewide assessments (Hatcher & Waguespack, 2004). Despite this legislation, educators struggle to develop accommodation policies that are perceived as fair and do not create "unfair advantages" for students with disabilities, meaning that students with disabilities are often seen to be getting a "leg up" by receiving extra time or other modifications. Surprisingly, there is a dearth of research documenting best practices in the area of accommodations and modifications. Indeed, there is controversy regarding the efficacy and presentation of assessment modifications, particularly extended time on tests. The controversy is whether these accommodations are over prescribed, particularly in certain socio-economic classes (Lovett, 2012). I will explore these topics in greater detail below.

COMMON ACCOMMODATIONS PROVIDED IN THE CLASSROOM

Certain accommodations are provided for almost all students with neurocognitive challenges. These are typically grouped into four categories:

1. Presentation of test items and classroom material. For example, the teacher may repeat the directions for an assignment or test, or he or she may read

the directions aloud. In addition, a modified response sheet might be provided for the students who may have difficulty with a Scantron (response sheet that requires students to fill in the bubbles on the sheet).

2. Response of the student to the test questions or classroom material. To illustrate, a student might be allowed to mark his or her answers in the booklet rather than use the scantron. In addition, the student might be allowed to use reference aids, such as a calculator or classroom notes, to complete the test or assignment.
3. Setting of the test. The test might be given in a separate room and special lighting may be provided.
4. Timing/scheduling of the test or assignment. In this case, the student might receive extended time or be allowed to take frequent breaks.

In addition to the above categories, students with disabilities may require general modifications in the learning environment. For example, they may need to sit near the teacher or get up and move about the classroom. In addition, they may benefit from previewing the events in the classroom; for example, they can get access to the curriculum ahead of time and learn some of the concepts so that they are better prepared when they encounter the concepts in the classroom.

Reading Accommodations

Accommodations are also tailored to the student's specific disability. For students with dyslexia, it may be useful to provide the student with the summary and vocabulary ahead of time, as previewing content can facilitate comprehension. In addition, graphic organizers, such as markers and sticky notes, can be used to arrange important text. Graphic organizers are an important tool as they focus the student on the most important material, facilitate comprehension, and cut down on the required amount of reading. Further, large print text facilitates reading as it enhances visual processing. Providing an audio version of the material can also be helpful for students with dyslexia, as they may have difficulty comprehending the material in a visual format. Lastly, the use of mnemonic devices (memory techniques) can facilitate retention in students with poor working memory. For example, an acronym such as "Roy G. Biv" can be used to help students remember the colors of the rainbow.

Math Accommodations

For students with dyscalculia, it might be helpful to allow the use of a calculator as these students may have trouble memorizing basic numerical facts. This will also enable them to solve math problems more accurately and efficiently. Highlighting key words in word problems can also be helpful as it reduces confusion and allows the student to focus on problem solving. Further, providing clear and well-defined worksheets facilitates comprehension and focus. Additionally, extra-large graph sheets can help compensate for poor visual processing and organization. Lastly, highlighting the arithmetic signs, such as addition and subtraction, can also direct the students' focus and cut down on careless errors.

Language Accommodations

For students with language-based learning disabilities, the suggested accommodations include use of visual or tactile aids as well as repetition and reinforcement of auditory material. Students can compensate for their auditory challenges with visual material, such as sheets and graphic organizers. Hands-on materials such as "manipulatives" for math (e.g., cubes and tiles) provide an experiential learning format which lessens students' dependence on verbal directions or lectures to understand the material. Use of written notes or outlines similarly reduces reliance on auditory information. Additionally, use of pre-selected oral cues (such as key words that have been reviewed and discussed) or repetition of key material improves comprehension and retention. Requiring the student to repeat or write down important information similarly helps compensate for poor auditory recall and comprehension. Lastly, recording the lecture is very helpful when the student is presented with an overwhelming amount of auditory information. They can either refer back to the notes or listen to the lecture again in order to fully grasp the material.

Writing Accommodations

When students have difficulty with writing, a designated notetaker can be provided so that the student does not need to take notes and listen at the same time and can focus on listening to facilitate comprehension. Access to the notes, either a fellow student's or the teacher's, can be essential to helping these learners review the material, thus enhancing recall. The teacher can also have the student answer questions orally instead of responding in writing. Frequently, use of a laptop is critical, particularly with students with handwriting challenges. In addition, use of Spell Check and Grammarly software improves the quality of the written work and helps avoid unfair penalties for students with writing disorders. Students may also benefit from use of a software program for outlining that will help with the organizational flow of their essays.

Scheduling Flexibility

For students with slowed processing speed, scheduling flexibility is often used. The school can offer more time to complete assignments, shorter assignments that cover the same work, shorter work periods, and more frequent breaks. Extended time can be a game changer as students have the opportunity to showcase their best work without being penalized for their slowed processing speed. A clinical anecdote illustrates this accommodation.

A bright, verbal tenth grader consistently received lower grades on her math tests and assignments because she failed to complete them on time. She found herself avoiding the assignments because they took so much time and then ended up staying up late into the night to complete her work. When given the opportunity to complete fewer problems and receive extra time on tests, her grades dramatically improved, her sleep habits returned to normal, and she began enjoying doing homework.

Attendance Flexibility

Flexibility with class attendance is another useful tool. This accommodation is widely used for students with neurocognitive challenges, both when they feel overwhelmed or need more time to complete an assignment, and thus need to skip a class to finish it. In addition, as neurocognitive challenges often give rise to depression and anxiety (see Chapter 3), this accommodation is most helpful when students need to take a "mental health" day or are not able to attend class due to psychiatric reasons. A clinical anecdote illustrates this accommodation:

A colleague commented that she worked with a student who had failed his first semester due to significant mental health and neurocognitive challenges. Specifically, he frequently missed classes and was unable to complete assignments on time. He was a bright, academically capable young adult but would lose so many points for missing class or handing in assignments late that he was unable to pass his classes. Upon returning to college, the learning center coordinator advocated for him to receive extended time on assignments and tests and attendance flexibility. These two accommodations proved greatly effective for this patient, and he was able to remain in college and pass all his classes as he was no longer penalized for inconsistent attendance or handing in assignments late (Ahola, 2022, personal communication).

ACCOMMODATIONS SPECIFIC TO COLLEGE-LEVEL COURSEWORK

The number of college programs for the learning disabled has increased since the late 1970s; In fact, 9 percent of incoming college students are labeled with some sort of disability (Henderson, 1999). Further, college presents unique academic and social demands that tap the student's strengths and weaknesses (Ryan & Heikkil, 1988). Thus, accommodations on the college level are a prominent issue for college educators.

Transitioning to an independent learning environment is challenging for all students but most challenging for students with neurocognitive deficits. College students are expected to multitask and be responsible for food, laundry, and the cleanliness of their room—in addition to classes and social life (Margalit & Shulman, 1986; Vogel, 1987). These demands can be overwhelming and may lead to compromised academic or emotional functioning. Moreover, deficits in reading, writing, and attention in the young adult may vary in intensity, duration, and frequency compared with the way they manifested in childhood (Alley et al., 1983).

As college-age students are expected to perform significantly more independently as compared with high school students, they often require accurate, detailed information regarding course expectations before selecting classes or majors (Seelig, 1987). Likewise, they may benefit significantly from recording the lectures and attending study groups (Mangrum & Strichart, 1984). In addition, access to notes is essential to accommodate those students who have difficulty listening and writing at the same time or who demonstrate expressive writing deficits (Decker et al., 1985).

Sweener et al. (2013) report that there is wide variability in the types of accommodations that were considered acceptable to faculty and students. Some college professors were rejecting of any accommodations, while others typically approved of extended time but did not allow access to notes whereas other faculty members were supportive of all accommodations that were recommended for these students. A clinical anecdote illustrates these issues:

> Working with a college student with Nonverbal Learning Disorder, I encouraged her to request extended time for her exams and access to notes. Although most professors were helpful, she encountered one professor who said that they never allowed anyone to have extended time or access to notes. This was extremely distressing and stressful for the student who wanted to drop the class. We devised a plan and emailed the coordinator of disability services asking her to intervene with this professor. With support for the coordinator, extended time was granted, and my patient felt that she could continue with the class.

In addition, many students encounter greater difficulty accessing accommodations in college compared to in high school, as they need to advocate for them on their own. There is not a built-in system for obtaining accommodations and college students no longer have their parents or other supportive figures to reinforce the need for such assistance. Therefore, therapists should be aware that these patients may require help in seeking out needed accommodations.

MODIFICATIONS

Accommodations do not change the standard to which the student is expected to perform; however, modifications are adjustments to assignments or tests that change the standard to what the test or assignment is supposed to measure (PACER Center, 2001). Thus, in contrast to accommodations, modifications can significantly alter the curriculum as well as the grading criteria. Here are some types of modifications in textbooks, curriculum, the classroom environment, and assignments that have been helpful for students with disabilities:

CURRICULUM

Modifications to the curriculum may include shorter assignments with a focus on key concepts, substitution of alternative projects for written assignments (such as poster projects), and presenting tests in an oral versus written format.

CLASSROOM ENVIRONMENT

Individualized rules for the student can be set regarding behavioral expectations and compliance with routines.

GRADING

It might be helpful to provide a partial grade based on individual progress or effort to help compensate for lack of comprehension of material. Further, the teacher can apply more weight daily work for a student who performs poorly on tests. Allowing students to revise their test and give them a grade on corrected work is very helpful for students with poor memory. Additionally, a pass-fail system for struggling students allows them to get credit for their work without being penalized by a poor grade on their transcript.

NEUROCOGNITIVE ASSISTIVE TECHNIQUES

In addition to accommodations and modifications, there are a plethora of diverse neurocognitive assistive techniques to facilitate academic progress for students with learning disorders. In general, these involve teaching specific skills, such as time management, organization of papers, and study skills, which are beneficial both for skills acquisition and goal attainment as well as the psychosocial skills of self-esteem and self-regulation (Richman et al., 2014). In addition, use of scaffolding or breaking the tasks down into small steps and using cues and prompts to facilitate task completion has been shown to be effective (Gersten et al., 1986.)

Direct instruction or explicit teaching has been shown to be an effective method with learning disabled students in a review of the literature (Adams & Engleman, 1991). Direct instruction includes goal-oriented lessons, corrective feedback, and opportunity for practice (Adams & Carmine, 2003). Teaching in short and intense spurts, making sure the students are engaged and on task, breaking down the steps, and providing opportunity for practice are critical elements of direct instruction (Joyce and Weil, 2004).

Further, there are specific techniques and strategies appropriate for each disorder's distinct challenges.

Assistive Techniques for Specific Disorders

Attentional Difficulties

Students with Attention Deficit Disorder often demonstrate poor executive functioning, manifesting in disorganization and impulsivity. Thus, teaching executive functioning skills can be essential for these students, both for their academic performance and emotional well-being (Parker et al., 2011). Specific examples include introducing students to a system of organizing papers and backpacks, helping them learn to use a planner to improve time management, and teaching general study skills to improve academic performance. In addition, a meta cognitive approach, in which students are helped to understand, monitor, and regulate their own cognitive processes, helps the students develop into effective and efficient learners (Thompson & Thompson, 1988; Flavell, 1979).

Modifications to the environment can include ensuring sufficient space to freely move around, assigning tasks that entail a great deal of movement, and providing a choice of seating that includes bouncy balls or chairs with sensory stimulation. In addition, fidget objects help focus and reduce anxiety.

Dyslexia

Students with reading disorders benefit from direct instruction and an individualized reading program, such as Orton-Gillingham (Ritchey et al., 2006) or the Wilson Method (Stebbins et al., 2012). More specific skills include phonic drills, that is, repetition and review of phonic rules and skills to improve sight vocabulary and strengthen the ability to attack unfamiliar words. Reading comprehension is facilitated by helping readers use context cues, that is, drawing on past information to understand the material and asking inferential questions, such as, "What is the main point of this passage? What do you think the characters were feeling in the passage?" Students are also helped to identify key concepts in the story. Annotation techniques are used as well, such as highlighting with markers, writing notes in the margins, and looking for common themes. Metacognitive techniques have also been shown to be extremely effective in facilitating academic progress, such that children are taught to use metacognitive strategies, that is, drawing on their experiences as an active learner, children are taught to be conscious of the strategies they are using as they perform academic tasks (Goldfus, 2012). For example, teaching the students to stop at the end of each paragraph to summarize what they are reading.

Modifications to the environment include making use of the numerous technological innovations that support reading and writing for individuals with learning disorders. Phones with speech-to-text conversion, computer programs such as spell check and Grammarly, and audiobooks are essential tools for school and work.

Dyscalculia

Students with math disorders benefit from direct instruction and an individualized math program such as the Singapore method (Preston, 2016). Breaking down the components, introducing manipulatives (e.g., tiles and blocks), and teaching systematic techniques to attack multistep and word problems all facilitate numerical facility. Use of adapted calculators (calculators that are color coded or "speak"), are also useful for individuals with dyscalculia and nonverbal learning disorder.

Disorder of Written Expression

Students who struggle with expressive writing benefit from outlining techniques and the use of graphic organizers, which are concrete sheets of directions that break down the task of writing into discrete sequences, such as topic sentences that double as prompts for the introduction, as well as using supporting sentences, that is, material that supports the topic and conclusion. Using an outline with students is essential. These students require specific directions on the basic structures of writing paragraphs such as topic sentences, supporting sentences and concluding sentences (Scott & Vitale, 2003). Computer programs, such as Inspiration, Grammarly, and Spell Check, are great tools for these writers.

Nonverbal Learning Disorder

Clearly marking the classroom and school to aid in getting around easily compensates for poor sense of direction. Use of online tools such as calendars to help schedule improves organization and productivity.

Autism Spectrum Disorder

Students with autism spectrum disorder benefit from help in learning how to analyze and respond to inferential questions. Scaffolding and direct instruction help these students move beyond the literal interpretation of the text to engage in more nuanced and sophisticated reasoning. In addition, social coaching, using role play and structured exercises, can be very helpful in improving social skills (Gantman et al., 2012). For example, students may act out a social conflict, discuss the feelings of each character, and learn tools for negotiating conflict.

Modifications to the environment include reducing sensory overload by introducing dim lighting and soundproofing in the office or learning space to render the environment as quiet as possible (Acasrdo et al., 2019). Further, rooms with low lighting, low noise, no perfumes, and a variety of seating arrangements can enhance quality of life for these students (Kinnaer et al., 2016). When students feel overloaded by environments that intrude on their senses either by being too bright, too noisy, or permeated with odors, they can retreat to a low sensory room to recharge. Sensory rooms offer multi-sensory engagement, using lights, textures, colors, and sounds (Kinnaer et al., 2016) Noise-canceling headphones can help individuals with ASD negotiate noisy streets and environments. Other adaptations can include weighted blankets, the ability to take breaks as needed, and sensory objects such as fidget toys to help focus and quell anxiety. In addition, peer mentors are critically important to provide emotional and social support (Sarrett, 2017), particularly given these learners, often compromised social skills.

ARE ACCOMMODATIONS HELPFUL?

The use of accommodations and services has been correlated with increased academic success (Howe, 2013). Nonetheless, the literature on the efficacy of specific accommodations is sparse. One literature review found students with disabilities to exhibit the greatest score gains relative to non-disabled students when given extended time (Sireci et al., 2005). Similarly, a study on math test scores showed that testing accommodations reduced the testing deficits caused by a student's learning disability (Tavani, 2004).

Moreover, studies indicate that most students with disabilities feel they need more academic support than what they are currently receiving in school, particularly in the areas of reading, writing, and completing homework (Sikirca et al., 2015). Students who were identified as needing the highest level of accommodations also had the highest level of school absence, suggesting a poor fit between the school and the student (Yngve et al., 2019). In college, students indicated that they found it necessary to continue using services and accommodations and they needed particular support with writing (Hadley, 2007, Allarakhia, 2017).

However, there is significant controversy about which accommodations are most useful, as no one accommodation has proven to be universally effective. There is no "one size fits all" in this area; thus, there is debate regarding efficacy for various populations (Fuchs et al., 2005). For example, test accommodations for children with ADHD have had mixed results, as many of these children do not benefit from extended time (Pritchard et al., 2016). A careful examination of the data indicated that there needs to be a differentiation between children with ADHD who are and are not impulsive, as impulsive children tend to fly through their work, make careless errors, and are often the first student to hand in their paper. Alternatively, children with ADD who demonstrate slow speed, difficulty with retrieving information, and "spaciness" benefit from extended time as it gives them the necessary opportunity to complete and review their work.

In contrast, extended test time for students with dyslexia is extremely effective and has a scientific rationale. Powerful neurobiological evidence indicates that people who are dyslexic read by a different pathway, one that takes more time. The fast-paced, automatic neural circuit is not available to individuals with dyslexia so they must take a secondary, slower pathway that will eventually allow them to decipher the printed word but at a cost of additional time (The Yale Center for Dyslexia and Creativity, 2017). As Sally Shaywitz said in *Overcoming Dyslexia*, "Dyslexia robs a person of time; accommodations return it" (Shaywitz, 2004).

CULTURAL CONCERNS

Another area of controversy involves the possible cultural bias of accommodations and the unequal access to them based on wealth and income. Testing accommodations are particularly controversial as it is feared that they could lead to higher test scores, which might be an unfair advantage, particularly in terms of college admissions. The *New York Times* found that students in the wealthiest 20 percent of schools were almost twice as likely as students in the poorest 20 percent of schools to receive 504 plans—the plans that provide a diagnosis and recommendations such as extended time (Royer & Randall, 2012). How does wealth lead to these high rates of disability identification and accommodations? Wealthier parents are more involved in their child's education and are more likely to pay for independent, private assessment (Calarco, 2018, Roberts, 2012). Thus, advantaged students receive possibly inappropriate accommodations that further contribute to higher test scores.

On the other hand, when disadvantaged children receive accommodations, it may prevent them from receiving adequate training in academic, organizational, and coping/emotional skills (Lovett, 2021). The staff may be inclined to give accommodations that would "solve" the problems as a "quick fix," rather than taking the time to help the child to learn the underlying skills.

Phillips (1994) suggested asking several questions to determine whether an accommodation is warranted:

1. Would the accommodation benefit nondisabled students as well?
2. Can the student with the disability adapt to standard conditions [with the aid of the accommodation]?

When the answer to the first question is yes, we should consider whether the accommodation is an unfair performance booster. When the answer to the second question is yes, the accommodation is warranted.

EMOTIONAL RESPONSES AND BARRIERS TO RECEIVING ASSISTIVE TECHNIQUES

Students often have intense emotional responses to receiving academic accommodations and support. Common reactions include feelings of shame, guilt, inadequacy, and discomfort. It is important that clinicians attend to the emotional effects of receiving academic support as they can lead students to avoid these services and consequently underperform academically. A major reason why students often might not utilize services is concern about peer reaction, as elicited in a survey of students with disabilities (Baker & Scanlon, 2016; Trammel & Hathaway, 2007). Students feel uncomfortable with their peers knowing that they need help and therefore are reluctant to request accommodations. A typical concern is that being pulled out of class for services or assessment is humiliating and the students feel "singled out." The stigma of not fitting in is particularly potent, as children are highly attuned to their social standing among peers, and fear of losing social status is a key motivator in school. In their survey on student perspectives on accommodations, Baker & Scanlon (2016) noted that students feel "embarrassed, weird and awkward" when receiving academic supports. They do not want peers to think they are "dumb, don't get it or could only succeed with accommodations." Fairness was another major concern. Peers will often express jealousy and complain that it is not fair that the special needs student gets more time or other types of help. This negative feedback further undermines the students' ability to feel comfortable receiving accommodations. A case example illustrates these conflicts.

> Leslie, an articulate young adult with significant attention, learning, and psychiatric challenges, successfully applied for extended time on her papers for graduate school. However, she expressed acute feelings of shame as her peers did not receive the same accommodations and she was worried she was coming across as "bratty, privileged and Special Education." We discussed her feelings of stigma and inadequacy in relation to her early traumatic experiences in school.

In a survey conducted by Marshak et al. (2010) on barriers to college students accessing accommodations, they noted that students might not utilize disability services due to identity issues, the desire to avoid negative social reactions, insufficient knowledge, and the perceived low quality and usefulness of services. Firstly, identity issues were prominent. The students want to feel self-sufficient; they want to shed their stigmatized identity in high school and not have to integrate the disability into their college identity. As college is a time of exploration and separation, it is reasonable that students want to be independent. Nonetheless, it often takes great effort to do so, and they may lose academic points as they struggle without needed support. Secondly, the desire to avoid their stigmatized high school identity is crucial. College is a time for self-invention and a fresh start for most students, so many students with disabilities want to shed their previous challenges and live their new lives like "normal" students. In addition, they are worried their peers might resent them for this "special treatment," and do not want to be singled out.

They would like to fit in, an understandable desire. Thirdly, students feel guilty about using accommodations, that they are not being "fair" to their peers. These themes are especially important as college students with learning disabilities who do not receive needed accommodations and support are at risk for failing classes and dropping out of college. Indeed, a review of the literature indicated that many such college students do not make use of their accommodations (Ferrell & Marshak, 2004; Jackson & Ferrell, 2000).

In my practice, I have found that college-age patients are more resistant to asking for services and therefore often "crash and burn" freshman year. I focus on helping my patients feel comfortable asking for accommodations. Accommodations do reduce anxiety, but it is important to understand the specific nature of the accommodations and how to help the student resolve their often-conflicted feelings about them (Lovett & Leja, 2013). Two case examples illustrate this phenomenon:

Jake, a bright, verbal 18-year-old with learning, attention, and psychiatric deficits, went away to college after successfully mainstreaming at a private high school that offered a great deal of academic support. Although Jake had received accommodations and support since he was 5 years old, he decided to be "independent" and did not request any services at school. He also elected not to take his ADD medication. Jake fell behind in his work and needed to take medical leave at the end of the semester. He also became severely depressed during the semester. Upon his return home, he spoke with me, his therapist, about how ashamed he feels about receiving accommodations and support. He confided that he feels dumb, inferior to his friends, and incompetent. We understood together how these feelings contributed to his refusal to receive services and began to strategize for the fall to create an effective academic plan for him.

Leslie, a bright, verbal young adult with Nonverbal Learning Disorder (mentioned in previous chapters) went to a different city for graduate school after a successful college experience where she lived with her parents and received support. Despite having received services and accommodations since kindergarten, she decided not to apply for accommodations in graduate school. She shared that she did not want to feel different from her peers, she was worried about what her peers and teachers would think of her, and was overwhelmed by the administrative process to procure accommodations. She then was unable to complete her research papers on time and needed to get extensions. Her feelings of shame regarding need for support interfered directly with her ability to complete her coursework.

TEACHER ROLES

Understanding the role of the teacher is crucial because they are generally the ones on the front lines administering the accommodations. Teachers often harbor misconceptions about accommodations that prevent them from providing accessible accommodations (Sniatecki et al., 2015). They are more likely to either deny or be skeptical about the existence of neurocognitive challenges in the students. Teachers are also more likely to provide accommodations if they can be easily administered to a range of students rather than a unique individual (Vallecorsa et al., 2000). Teachers are also concerned about fairness to the other students (Maccini & Gagnon, 2006). However, teachers do not find providing instructional accommodations as challenging (Scanlon & Baker, 2012). This case example illustrates the complexity of getting the school to provide adequate accommodations.

Sally, a bright tenth grader with dyslexia (mentioned in Chapter 2) was mainstreamed from a special education school to a private school that provided a great deal of support. She received extended time, special education instruction, and allowances for spelling. However, at the end of the year, finals were administered as an in-class essay. This type of testing was punitive for Sally as, due to her poor working memory and severe dyslexia, she could not construct a coherent, well-organized essay with proper syntax and grammar. Her mother, who proofread her papers, commented that the word choices were often so misspelled you could not figure out their meanings unless she told you what she meant. The examiner asked the school to allow Sally access to notes during the test so she could write out her essays ahead of time, have the chance to make revisions with support, and then write them during the test. The school refused, citing concerns about fairness or the other students. We explained that this testing method hit Sally squarely in her learning disability and it was unfair for her to be assessed in this manner. The school said they would take it under consideration.

In a 2010 survey study, Scanlon & Baker (2010) identified that issues related to interactions with professors were among the most significant challenges to accessing services in college. Several students were confronted with situations in which a professor would not fully believe that the student truly had a disability (even though documentation was provided) or would not believe that the student's disability was the reason for missing class. Other students encountered situations in which they would ask the professor for copies of the class lecture or overhead slides, but the professor would refuse.

Allarkhia (2017) conducted a survey of students who receive academic accommodations and found that faculty is often resistant to accommodations. Training for faculty was recommended so that the teachers should understand that accommodations are not a "luxury" but are mandated by federal law. Moore et al. (2020) recommended three aspects of disability inclusion for teachers: first, to lead with humility (i.e., the trainer should be respectful of the teacher's expertise), second, to build authentic relationships and, third, to solve problems with consensus building. Consensus building is a method of collaborating with the teachers, educating them regarding the issues and eliciting solutions from them.

Focused trainings are essential to educate college faculty about learning disabilities and how to help students with this hidden handicap. Historically, support for students with special needs have been built through in-service training, direct consolation, independent reading, and advanced coursework for teachers in K–12 (Ryan & Heikilla, 1988). This approach needs to be also applied to higher education as increased awareness will lead to delivery of more effective accommodations.

SELF-ADVOCACY

But faculty training alone will not ensure that college students will receive the necessary accommodations. According to the National Center for Learning Disabilities (NCLD), 7 percent of college students who identify as needing an accommodation for a learning disability do not inform the college they attend of this requirement (Horowitz et al., 2017). Not disclosing this information can lead to a low rate of college completion (Hotowitz et al., 2017). As noted above, research in this area attributes non-disclosure to low self-esteem, fear of being perceived as lazy or unintelligent, wanting to create an identity beyond their disability, and the general stigma regarding a learning disability (Gerber, 2011).

Effective methods to help students self-advocate have been extensively investigated. Research shows that high school students have limited ability to advocate and use their accommodations (Byrnes, 2008). For students to use accommodations effectively, they must understand their accommodation needs and be able to communicate about them with teachers and peers (Milsom & Hartley, 2005). However, when students learned skills of self-advocacy, their use of accommodations improved significantly (Shogren et al., 2012). Further, high school seniors who were educated about their accommodations reported feeling more confident about achieving academic success (Wood et al., 2010). These interventions have also been successful on a college level as a self-advocacy intervention facilitated Black college students with intellectual disabilities to request academic accommodations (Brendli et al., 2021).

METACOGNITIVE INTERVENTIONS

Metacognitive intervention helps students become better learners by teaching them to reflect upon their cognitive strategies—in effect, to think about thought. Specific strategies include rehearsal (repeating new information), elaboration (summarizing, paraphrasing), and organization (e.g., note taking). Also, techniques such as working from end-states backwards and estimation of task difficulty represent strong strategies for planning and problem solving (Pintrich, 2002). These techniques have been shown to be effective in working with students with LDs. For example, students with NVLD who were taught problem-solving skills in a sequenced manner improved their math skills, as they were able to transfer these skills to master math concepts. This sequence went from concrete, to semi-concrete, to abstract instruction. For example, the instruction begins with use of physical manipulatives such as blocks, then progresses to visual images, and then to solving programs with the formal symbols of mathematics. Thus, the students understood the algebraic concepts before being asked to memorize facts and logarithms. (Maccini & Hughes, 2000). Such strategies are applicable to all academic skills and subjects as they help the student understand how to be a student—that is, learn concepts and apply them to problems.

COMMON MISCONCEPTIONS

To maximize the efficacy of accommodations and support self-advocacy among students and parents alike, it is critical to address misconceptions about academic accommodations. I have noticed several common ones in my work with students, teachers, and parents. Firstly, the idea of accommodations as a crutch is often mentioned. Similarly, there is a fear that receiving accommodations will stunt the student's ability to learn, implying that there is only one way to learn the material. If you are getting accommodations or support, somehow you are not going about it correctly and will not be able to succeed. The other misconception is that the accommodations are not applicable to the real world; thus, in order to help the student function normally, they should be treated like "everybody else." Of course, the students themselves want to be treated as "normal" and are deeply worried about stigma.

I use the analogy of an "invisible wheelchair" to help people understand the fallacy of these misconceptions. Just as we would not expect wheelchair-bound individuals to walk and would not penalize them for this disability, we cannot expect the individual with neurocognitive impairment to operate as a neurotypical student. "Leveling the playing field" is another useful metaphor, to convey the idea that accommodations allow the student to participate on an equal footing with neurotypical students rather than creating an unfair advantage.

HOW CAN THE THERAPIST HELP?

Firstly, the therapist's role is to help the patient understand the need for and benefit of accommodations. Explaining the patient's neurocognitive style and delving into the nuts and bolts of how the accommodations will be helpful is essential to this process. Secondly, the therapist needs to be mindful that the patients have complex feelings regarding accommodations; they may feel encouraged, relieved, and supported, but they may also feel they are "cheating" or are "frauds." In addition, they may feel stigmatized and singled out by teachers and peers; thus, the therapist needs to help dispel these misconceptions and encourage the patient to advocate effectively. Lastly, the therapist can teach self-advocacy to patients using psychoeducation and role playing. McGahee (2021) taught self-advocacy very successfully to patients with learning disabilities with the use of role play. A case example illustrates this technique:

> Leslie, the young adult with NVLD mentioned above, needed to receive extra time on tests in college but was scared to ask for help from the disability office. We role-played her leaving my office, then returning to knock on the door and ask for the accommodation. We also explored her feelings of anxiety and fear of rejection as related to early experiences of bullying and stigma for being taken out of class for services. Leslie was soon able to successfully self-advocate for extended time.

In sum, receiving accommodations and modifications is an essential ingredient in facilitating academic success. In order for students to feel comfortable receiving accommodations they need to explore their feelings of shame, guilt, inadequacy, and fear of stigma. The therapist can facilitate this process by countering misconceptions, using role-play, and helping the student advocate for support.

Chapter Five

Understanding the Impact of Neuropsychological Testing on Patients with Neurocognitive Challenges

Integrating Test Results into the Treatment

Patients with attention and learning issues, as well as autism spectrum disorder, will most likely have been assessed multiple times during their academic and/or professional careers. Understanding the emotional impact of the testing on the patient as well as the family is essential for intervention with this population. Further, the test results can be extremely useful during the treatment to help patients and their families understand the diagnosis, advocate successfully for services and accommodations, and dispel painful misconceptions about their deficits. This chapter will explore the impact of assessment and provide specific recommendations on how to use the test results most effectively in treatment. I will begin by discussing the impact on the patient and families and how to work with these issues.

PSYCHOLOGICAL IMPACT ON PATIENTS AND FAMILIES

Impact on the Patient

This section will focus mainly on children as they comprise the majority of testing cases, although the impact on adults will also be discussed. Children may find both assessment and receiving test feedback quite painful. Siegel (1987) proposed that children may dread the exposure of their weaknesses in the testing situation. They may feel caught, thinking they had been fooling everybody about their challenges, but now need to "fess up." Many bright children with learning/attentional difficulties are aware of their limitations and have been consciously disguising them for fear of exposure and embarrassment. They can be resistant to addressing areas of weakness and feel overwhelmed by the services recommended. Children often come up with their own explanations for their difficulties or internalize the way caregivers have responded to them. They tell themselves "I'm stupid, I can't do it," and so on. They may feel committed to these self-perceptions and reluctant to embrace other ways of understanding challenges.

Alternatively, children may feel relieved that the adults are collaborating on a plan to address their difficulties. They may feel understood for the first time around academic, social, and emotional difficulties. Self-esteem may improve as they let go of toxic ideas, replacing them with more helpful models of understanding how their minds work. Thus, child therapists must keep in mind the diverse responses to testing and feedback and work actively to understand the child's responses and help them adjust to the diagnosis.

Adults may have similar responses to testing and feedback. They may feel relieved and understood by receiving a diagnosis and an analysis of their strengths and challenges. Alternatively, they may feel "caught out," exposed, and vulnerable. They may feel angry that their neurocognitive issues were not correctly addressed before adulthood and blame their parents or teachers for neglecting the etiology of their poor performance. When working with adults and exploring the impact of the testing and feedback, it is important to keep in mind how they may have experienced this significant life event as children if they were tested during childhood.

Impact of Assessment and Feedback on Parents

Assessment and feedback can have strong effects on parents as well as children, both therapeutic and painful (Bennett-Levy et al., 1994; Finn and Tonsager, 1997; Gorske, 2008; Hamilton et al., 2009). Human and Teglasi (1993) reported favorable changes in parents' self-reports following testing feedback, including an improved understanding of their child and improved parent-child relationships. Nonetheless, the information testers impart exposes the child's difficulties, which can be hard for parents to hear. The parents' anxiety about their child's future is often triggered and their wishes regarding the child may make it difficult to hear the feedback. When parents are able to voice their concerns, however, they can become more receptive to information about their children's challenges.

Parents may feel angry and distressed by the exposure of their child's challenges. They may also be overwhelmed by the steps required to address the issues. Additionally, parents often blame themselves and feel guilty about how they may have mistreated their children prior to neuropsychological testing, since they did not yet understand their children's challenges. Likewise, parents often express anger regarding prior consults that did not reveal their children's academic and psychological difficulties. For example, one mother on receiving feedback about her daughter's dyslexia expressed anger that the school and pediatrician did not previously uncover her daughter's challenges when the mother had discussed her concerns with them and that she had "wasted time" with ineffective reading techniques.

Shame is a particularly potent and often unexpressed emotion that parents can feel during the testing process. It can be experienced as a narcissistic injury to learn that one's child has neurocognitive and/or psychiatric difficulties (Fajardo, 1983). Parents may feel that the disability is a negative reflection on their own genes, parenting skills or abilities.

On the other hand, for many parents, diagnosis comes as a relief. Parents often experience many challenging years without understanding their child's difficulties and thus feel supported and empowered when they finally receive the correct diagnosis. On more than one occasion I have heard a parent exclaim, "I knew there was something wrong, but nobody would tell me what it was." Now better prepared to make informed decisions regarding interventions, schools, and services for their children, parents can feel hope and even excitement for the future. Moreover, they can finally understand and empathize with the child's learning and/or emotional issues, which frequently improves the parent-child relationship. In some cases, the child's diagnosis resonates with parents who then express a wish to be evaluated themselves. A common parental reaction is, "I bet if you tested me, you would find the same thing!"

Paul, an engaging 9-year-old boy, was referred due to significant academic difficulties. Testing revealed deficient language skills with low average to average visual-spatial skills. As a result, academic skills were significantly below grade level. The boy had been previously assessed by the Board of Education with minimal services recommended to him. The parents had been very distressed regarding his low scores that reflected his language-based learning disability. I explained the etiology of his low scores as related to his struggles with verbal tasks and guided them in obtaining a special education placement for their son. The family expressed relief regarding the results and recommendations.

In sum, when working with children who have been recently diagnosed, including the family, the work is essential to facilitate awareness and ensure that the child is receiving appropriate support. Likewise, adult patients with a childhood history of learning challenges can benefit from discussing their family's response during their childhood to their testing, diagnosis, and need for services.

I will now address how to discuss test results with the patients and families in order to ensure that the test results are understood by patients and their families. Ideally, the therapist can use the test results to dispel these misconceptions and to facilitate self-esteem and confidence.

INTERPRETING DATA TO PATIENTS

Testing feedback is generally provided by the tester. However, the therapist often reinforces the findings, provides context for the results, and supports the patients' newfound appreciation of their strengths and challenges. It is helpful to encourage clients to listen to the interpretation of the results rather than focusing on the numbers. Using numbers and data points to describe the results can upset and overwhelm patients, as the data, if taken alone, can be misleading or confusing. Patients and families should also be encouraged to focus on recommendations and summaries, as this provides actionable information for problem solving.

Feedback to children should not include any numbers but should focus on their specific strengths and challenges. Further focus should be placed on strategies they can employ to help compensate for areas of weakness. For example, children who present with auditory processing disorder can sit in front of the class, do homework in a quiet environment, and use earplugs in noisy places. Similarly, feedback with adults should focus on solutions to the presenting problem. For example, modifications to the workplaces, concrete suggestions of intervention, and accommodations.

Allowing the children to read the entire report is not optimal, as they can often become overwhelmed with the information and feel criticized. However, if an adolescent or young adult insists, they should be encouraged to read the report with the therapist present, which allows for elucidation of questions. The concerns are most often around low scores, which can be usually explained by helping the patient realize that the score reflects the impact of their difficulties on their performance and is not a reflection of their intelligence.

What does a clinician do when the child has low scores as a result of global intellectual disabilities? Often children are referred due to significant neurocognitive deficits. If that is the case, it is very important to instruct the parent not to share the scores with the child. The parent should always focus on the areas of strength and encourage the child to feel positively about his or her skills. Often, coming up with an appropriate school placement is essential in these cases to provide support for the child.

COMMON MISCONCEPTIONS

Dispelling misconceptions surrounding children's problems is one of the most challenging but rewarding aspects of therapy. Untangling the neurocognitive and psychiatric underpinnings of children's underperformance and maladaptive behavior at home and in school provides clarity and understanding. For example, with feedback, parents can understand that attention deficit disorder with hyperactivity (ADHD) can cause children to space out and not hear teachers or parents. This does not mean that they are oppositional. Likewise, an anxious/avoidant response to learning difficulties can look like procrastination or poor motivation. Nonetheless, helping the children and their families understand that the child is not "stupid, lazy, or bad" is complicated and requires time (Kelly and Ramundo, 2014).

Parents are sometimes suspicious of the diagnoses and the recommended services. They may fear that the diagnosis itself and the recommended supports will become crutches that will further limit or even disable their children. Parents may say, "Oh, he just needs discipline. If we tell him he has ADHD, he will use it as an excuse to not do his homework." They may be concerned that tutoring or medication will take away the child's independence, because taking advantage of these types of support will mean that he will not be "doing the work himself." Analogies such as an "invisible wheelchair" and "eyeglasses," convey how learning deficits are as valid as observable physical deficits and stress that the child is receiving needed services. The aim, therefore, should be to facilitate success while acknowledging the child's limitations. The therapist can use the test results to identify realistic goals and expectations based on the child's areas of strength as well as challenges.

REJECTION OF THE TEST RESULTS

What may seem crystal clear to the clinician is often misunderstood by the family. At times, it may seem like the clinician and family are speaking two different languages. What does the therapist do when the feedback is perceived as negative or when patients and families disagree or reject the diagnosis and/or recommendations? This issue is rarely discussed in the literature but often comes up in the consulting room. Most often the negativity reflects anxiety and a wish to avoid bad news. The therapist can interrupt this negative cycle by allying with the parents. The therapist can say, "We don't need to put a label on your child. We just need to understand what's going on and figure out how to help." What is aimed for is a meeting of minds with a focus on problem solving. In addition, the clinician should inquire more about the concerns in order to understand why the parent may be rejecting the test results.

The mother of a 9-year-old boy received feedback that her son is highly intelligent, with ADHD and anxiety. To my surprise, the mother was highly resistant to this feedback and was distressed that her son was not diagnosed with autism spectrum disorder, as he had been previously. I struggled to understand her concerns and realized that she was worried that her son would stop receiving the free services that the Department of Education was providing for him. I set up another meeting with her to address her concerns. With the additional diagnosis of auditory processing disorder, confirmed by an audiologist to whom I referred her, the mother felt more confident that her son would continue receiving services.

It is not simple to help the family navigate the thicket of their emotional responses at the same time as their practical concerns. Parents are vulnerable to feeling inferior or judged by the examiner, and it is important for the therapist to establish him or herself as a "like subject" (i.e., someone to whom the parents can relate) in order both to build an alliance and reduce the asymmetry of the testing situation. Helping the family understand that they are not alone and that many other families struggle with similar issues can take the sting out of the data and replace some of these negative feelings with feelings of hope and optimism.

What does a therapist do when the parent seems committed to the idea of the child being defective, lazy, or stupid rather than having neurocognitive or psychiatric issues? It can be frustrating and upsetting to the clinician to hear parents blame the child and/or reject feedback that could be useful. Maybe the blaming functions as a rejection of the deficit and a hope that the child can change rather than an acceptance of the diagnosis. Taking a long-term view of the situation can often be helpful to the clinician. Understanding that this is a process and allowing the ideas to percolate with the family can help counter parents' resistance and give them room to assimilate test results gradually. As above, if the therapist can find a way to allow parents to express their concerns, this can diminish parental resistance to the diagnosis.

DIVISION WITHIN THE FAMILY

Parents often have different views about their child—this is more frequently the case when they are separated or divorced. It is important for the clinician to maintain a neutral stance and support each parent. This is a balancing act that may involve separate sessions and a great deal of tact. There may be a power struggle between the parents regarding who is right and who sees the situation clearly. The therapist needs to negotiate the conflict without leaving one parent feeling blamed or dismissed.

Consultation about a 25-year-old young woman who demonstrated serious issues with daily living skills revealed that the parents differed in their concerns. The mother discussed her concern that the daughter receives around-the-clock supervision, as she would easily get lost and appeared to be unaware of her surroundings. The father was concerned that the daughter was receiving too much support and using it as a crutch. He wanted the daughter to achieve independence. In my consultation, I stressed that each parent had a valuable contribution and commitment to their daughter's success. I affirmed that the daughter's neurocognitive impairments created difficulties with time management, directions, and self-care, and did necessitate intensive supervision. Concomitantly, I commented on her intelligence and high academic aptitude, and affirmed her abilities in the areas of reading and writing. The parents began to collaborate more effectively as the mother felt supported in advocating care for her daughter, and the father was able to absorb more information about the daughter's challenges when they were presented along with areas of strength.

Working With the School

School Observations

To best help the child, it is often necessary to integrate test results with information gathered from the school and other professionals. Children's teachers, tutors, and other professionals are valuable sources of information and should be consulted by therapists. A classroom observation can round out the picture and illuminate specifics of the child's behavior. It is valuable to observe children during a structured academic task as well as during unstructured times such as recess or lunch. Incorporation of this information into work with the family can enhance the therapeutic alliance with the parents. When the therapist can weave in anecdotal information about the child from these sources, the parents can better understand the test results and become more receptive to them.

An assessment of a preschool boy revealed a bright, verbal child with significant distractibility and a short attention span. When I observed him in the classroom, I noted his engagement with his peers, his love of building, and his motivation to please his teachers. During conversations with the teachers and parents, I relayed my observation that he was one of the first children to comply with the direction to stop playing and go to the rug for circle time. He sat on the rug and assumed a yoga pose, apparently attempting to regulate and focus. Although he was only able to sit in the circle and attend to the teacher for the first 10 minutes of the lesson, his motivation to please and to cooperate was impressive. The teachers and parents enjoyed the anecdote and told me that he was a "good boy" despite his difficulty complying with classroom routines and expectations. My observations about their son's behavior at circle time made these parents feel that I understood and was sympathetic toward their son. This greatly aided in their capacity to accept the test results.

School observations bring to light the child's strengths and weaknesses and pave the way to understanding the test results in a child's real-life setting. The clinician can use the observations to connect the dots for the parents and teachers and relate how the child's learning style and neurocognitive functioning impacts his or her behavior and productivity in the classroom. Additionally, observations conducted during recess and lunchtime highlight the child's social emotional functioning and often point to a need for intervention in those areas.

Feedback to the School

As the overwhelming majority of assessments of children are directly related to school performance, effectively working with school personnel is imperative for successful testing outcomes. What happens when the parent is reluctant to share information with the school? Parents often feel wary about how the school will respond to the results. They may feel concerned that the results might stigmatize their children. They may even worry that the school will expel the child. The therapist can encourage the parent to share information, explaining that the results will help the child to be better understood by teachers and receive needed accommodations.

Once the parent agrees to share the results with the school, how do you decide how best to present the feedback to the school's teachers and administration? Feedback to the school can be communicated in face-to-face meetings, phone consultations, and email. Each modality calls for different skills. A meeting with the therapist, parents, and school professionals can be extremely useful to help the school better understand the child and implement specific accommodations and interventions. The school psychologist, guidance counselor, learning specialist, and other support staff are often key participants in these meetings. Should the child be invited to attend the feedback meeting with the school? Older adolescents often benefit from attending the school meetings as they can experience firsthand the information that is presented to their teachers and can learn what they need to do to advocate for themselves. In many schools, adolescents are expected to arrange extended time on tests with their teachers. Clarifying the process with the student, parents, and teachers promotes effective follow up by the student.

For the younger child, explaining the etiology of behaviors is often the most valuable piece of the meeting. Children often say, "I won't," when they mean "I can't." They can get inexplicably upset, refuse to comply with rules or withdraw from tasks as a result of learning, attention, and psychiatric challenges. Deciphering behaviors and learning styles can be enlightening for teachers and guide them in appropriate interventions with the children. For example, a child who was refusing to complete math work was able to successfully respond to problems when the format of the worksheet was changed to accommodate his visual processing issues.

In another example, an assessment of a 10-year-old girl revealed significant learning issues, particularly in the area of reading. While she presented as a bright and verbal child, teachers reported behavioral difficulties such as tearfulness, distractibility, and lack of compliance with directions. Her mother consulted with me regarding these observations. When I asked for more specifics about when these behaviors occurred, it became clear that they tended to happen during reading instruction. The girl would become distressed, stop attending to class material, walk around the room and not be able to follow the curriculum presented in class. Her mother had not shared the test results with the school due to concern about the school labeling her daughter and attaching negative consequences to the information. She was worried her daughter would be asked to leave the school. I explained how the feedback would benefit the child by helping the teachers understand that she was distressed about her reading skills. When I conducted a phone feedback session with the school, the teachers began to accommodate the child's learning style by providing individualized instruction during that time. The child's behavior significantly improved.

Sometimes, however, it is the school administration or the teachers that have a rigid perspective on the child and have difficulty incorporating information from the testing about the child's learning style. For example, the teacher may feel the student is "unmotivated" and could really accomplish the work if he or she just "put in some effort." Thus, the school may not be receptive to implementing accommodations or modifications. The information may need to be conveyed over time and in as collaborative a manner as possible. The clinician can work directly with school personnel to understand their concerns and then help guide the parents regarding how best to work with the school. If the child is disruptive in class, the clinician can suggest different behavioral strategies. If the child is not advancing academically, it is useful to clarify expectations and ensure that the child can meet those standards. There are times that the child may require a different school placement. In these cases, the clinician can offer suggestions for a more appropriate school setting or refer the family to a school consultant.

The guiding principles are to address the questions and concerns professionals have about the student and provide clear recommendations for intervention. Always, the therapist needs to be mindful that the other team members may have different perspectives on the student and to find a way to communicate the test results effectively and respectfully.

An assessment of a 9-year-old boy revealed impaired reading comprehension due to an overly concrete and rigid learning style. He also evidenced anxiety and attention difficulties. A team approach was suggested that included tutoring in reading with a specialist, therapy and medication with a psychiatrist, and small group instruction in school. At the end of the school year a meeting was called with the parents, teachers, and school administrators to discuss progress and recommendations for the fall. During the meeting, confusion was voiced about the boy's erratic behavior and reading skills. The teacher offered an observation: "He can't work independently, and he can only finish a project when I sit with him." She felt this behavior was "emotional" and "volitional." I agreed that the student was anxious and impulsive and complimented the teacher on her ability to be supportive and reassuring.

I then explained that the student was not deliberately causing trouble or being overly demanding. Instead, his behaviors were the result of his neurocognitive difficulties; he had great difficulty organizing his thoughts, extrapolating information, and making inferences. He worked better with the teacher as he was receiving cues from her that compensated for his areas of difficulty. I showed the teacher how she was scaffolding him, that is, giving him sequential cues as she sat with him, and how he benefited from this structure. These insights facilitated better understanding of his learning style and improved the teacher's ability to work effectively with him.

Using the test results effectively in a school setting often requires parents and therapists to be forceful and insistent in advocating for services for the child. One mother commented, "When you told me my child needed resource room services, the Board of Education said 'no.' I was so convinced that you knew what was right for my child that I told them I am not leaving until my child gets those services. I got her into the resource room, and she flourished." For parents and therapists, having the confidence and know-how to advocate for the children and get them the services and accommodations they need is imperative in facilitating academic success.

A 10-year-old boy frequently wandered out of his classroom to complain to the principal about somatic or emotional concerns. Testing revealed that the student was missing basic writing skills and was leaving the classroom to avoid these tasks. The principal referred to the behavior as "manipulative." I explained that the student becomes overloaded and disorganized when presented with challenging work due to his learning difficulties. Several strategies were recommended including use of an iPad, dictation, and teacher support to help the student with his writing issues and indirectly to help him control his disruptive behavior. The teacher incorporated these techniques in working with the child, and the wandering behaviors subsided.

HOW CAN THE THERAPIST HELP THE CHILD AND FAMILY ASSIMILATE THE TEST RESULTS?

Because assimilating new information is difficult and requires time, it is helpful to offer several consultation sessions to help the family unpack the results and ensure that they fully understand the feedback. A typical scenario is a feedback session for the parents, then for the child, and then follow-up with a family feedback session. This aims to create a situation in which everyone is on the same page. Omitting the family feedback session can lead to conflicts within the family, as parents and child may insist that the tester offered different feedback. A family feedback session is crucial to ensure that parents and children hear the same information at the same time. The family session is also an opportunity to consolidate information, vent reactions to the testing and/or feedback, and provide practical suggestions and strategies.

Once the parent and child understand a diagnosis, the therapist is in a position to come up with recommendations that address the concerns. The therapist encourages the family to approach the recommendations as suggestions and empower the family to pick and choose among those recommendations that make sense for them as a family. Families often need to make decisions that directly impact the child such as choosing a new school and professionals to work with the child.

The therapist can check in with the parents to make sure that the information being provided makes sense to them, and request examples from them that either confirm or contradict the results. For example, children with

ADHD often have trouble complying with household routines and chores. This can be a good jumping off point for a family to begin to discuss the impact of the child's difficulties on family life. A common complaint is that the child does everything slowly and is delayed in leaving the house. When parents understand that the slowed speed is neurocognitive, they can begin to brainstorm strategies that will facilitate transitions. For example, use of a whiteboard in the child's room with a check-off list of items can jog the child's memory and eliminate the nagging that previously accompanied each morning. This will lead to a more relaxed start of the day.

WORKING WITH TESTERS

Sometimes, the tester also provides therapy; oftentimes, that is not the case. If the testing is performed by someone other than the therapist, the therapist needs to be able to collaborate with the tester effectively. This collaboration can be complicated by many factors. Does the tester have a different theoretical orientation than the therapist? Does the therapist have a different view of the child than the tester? Further, the potential for splitting within the family requires sophisticated clinical management. The therapist has ultimate clinical responsibility and all suggestions for treatment should be directed to the therapist. I often suggest a joint session with the parents and the tester, particularly if there are complicated treatment decisions to make. Use of statements such as "We are all on the same team," and making it clear how much the therapist respects the tester is instrumental in maintaining a productive working relationship with all parties.

CONCLUSIONS

Patients with attention and learning issues as well as autism spectrum disorder are frequently assessed as part of diagnosis and intervention. Test results can be used to improve understanding of the patient, facilitate self-confidence, and help advocate for support and accommodations. However, patients and families often have intense and complex emotional responses to test results, and therapists can greatly benefit from understanding the range and meaning of these responses to assessment and feedback.

Chapter Six

Treatment for Patients with Neurocognitive Impairments

An Integrated Approach

As discussed in Chapter 3, the psychosocial implications of neurocognitive impairments can be devastating for both children and their families. Briefly, individuals with learning and attention disorders often present with significant psychiatric symptoms including anxiety and depression. The root of these symptoms lies in the experience of academic and social failure stemming from their neurocognitive deficits. The repeated experiences of failure lead to painful feelings of frustration, disappointment, and pervasive problems with low self-esteem. Additionally, children with these deficits frequently face criticism from parents, teachers, and peers, leading to interpersonal conflict and internalized self-criticism. As adults, neurocognitive challenges may continue to interfere with academic, social, and professional functioning. In addition, adult patients with neurocognitive deficits harbor traumatic experiences of failure and frustration as children. Thus, it is crucial in treatment to address the psychological impact of these challenges.

Working with patients with learning and attention disorders requires a multifaceted approach, as there needs to be multiple foci: patients' neurocognitive deficits, the psychiatric symptoms that accompany these challenges, and the traumatic aspects of the patients' development due to their neurocognitive challenges and other people's responses to it—that is, parents, peers, and teachers. Clinical intervention should include psychoeducation and problem solving that helps the patients understand the neurocognitive underpinnings of their challenges, dispelling misconceptions about their learning disabilities, and coming up with effective strategies for their day-to-day difficulties. Psychodynamic/insight-oriented work comes into play when exploring the devastating emotional impact of the disorders. When working with adults, this involves helping them remember and recognize their feelings when dealing with this disorder in childhood. When working with children, the therapist is dealing with these issues in real time and is often called upon to advocate for the patient with the school, family or both.

The intervention comes in segments: psychoeducation about the learning disorder, exploration regarding the feelings accompanying this information, introduction of strategies to cope with the practical aspects of the disorder, exploration of the past experiences with the disorder, helping the patient experience all these feelings and, ultimately, facilitating their acceptance of their neurocognitive challenges and unique skill set. As patients progress, they painstakingly acquire a more integrated sense of self that encompasses understanding and acceptance of their neurodiversity. This complex and nuanced approach does not always proceed sequentially but is fluid and matches the patient's pace (Sorscher, 2021). Although I am describing these interventions as sequential, in treatment, the therapist may need to shift back and forth from one approach to another over time or even use all these techniques in one session.

These specific interventions shift the self-blame away from patients' global sense of self and onto a specific physical condition. This frees them to consider strategies for these challenges. Given the profound impact on the developing psyche, education about these deficits can take years to accomplish as the self-blame and negative self-image are deeply ingrained and can appear quite intractable. The patient and therapist often need to develop a shared vocabulary about the learning and/or attention deficits that feels tolerable for the patient. Relearning how to view oneself and reframing areas of challenge and frustration is a painful and incremental task that must be done in tandem with insight-oriented treatment as well as academic/professional support.

GENERAL TREATMENT TARGETS FOR EACH DISORDER

While all patients with neurocognitive challenges share struggles with self-acceptance and adaptation to their neurodiversity, there are also issues specific to each class of disorders. As a necessary first step, treatment aims to elucidate the etiology of and dispel misconceptions about each patient's disorder.

Learning Disorders

Individuals with nonverbal learning disorders are verbal and articulate and are seen as "flighty" or "needy" when they get lost or have difficulty performing visual-spatial tasks, such as reading diagrams or maps. In treatment, helping them understand that they have a real issue that is not "in their head" and has ramifications for their performance can be an uphill battle. Organization and time management challenges are also part of this disorder; thus, explicating the neurological etiology of these challenges is a crucial initial step to improving their skills.

Individuals with language-based learning disorders have difficulty expressing themselves; they are often tongue tied in social and academic situations. As core academic tasks such as reading and writing are significant areas of challenge, their self-esteem suffers, and they frequently describe themselves as "stupid." They can be seen as shy, oppositional, and non-communicative. Explaining the etiology of their academic and social issues is vital to improving self-esteem and rebuilding confidence. Once they understand that their communication and academic challenges are due to their learning issues, they are able to address them more effectively and their self-esteem improves.

Attention Disorders

Individuals with executive functioning disorder and ADD similarly suffer from misconceptions about their challenges. Their high level of distractibility and lack of focus makes it painful to initiate and complete academic tasks. In addition, they can inadvertently offend peers with their tangential conversation and disinhibited comments. They too often perceive themselves as lazy and stupid. Highlighting their areas of strength and emphasizing their abilities to adapt to their challenges facilitates self-confidence and productivity. Describing famous role models who have ADD and emphasizing their unique assets, such as creativity, high level of energy, ability to think "outside the box" and good risk-taking skills, helps improve self-esteem.

Autism Spectrum Disorder

Individuals with high functioning autism have the most significant challenges in social/interpersonal situations as they have difficulty understanding emotions, taking other people's perspectives, and responding to social nuances and cues. As such, they are often misperceived as "rude" or "oppositional." Understanding the neurocognitive underpinnings of their challenges and teaching them coping strategies in social situations facilitates their ability to initiate and sustain relationships. Role playing and providing scripts is exceptionally helpful because it provides them with a cognitive framework to execute appropriate social responses.

PSYCHOTHERAPY LITERATURE

We will now address the psychotherapy literature for neurodivergent individuals. There is support in the literature for diverse therapeutic approaches with this patient population. Both research and clinical studies support the efficacy of both medication and different psychotherapy approaches, including Cognitive Behavior Therapy (CBT), Dialectical Behavior Therapy (DBT), group therapy, parent training, and behavior modification. I will review some of the current studies documenting the efficacy of varied therapeutic approaches with each disorder and provide case examples for each approach.

PSYCHOEDUCATION

Psychoeducation is a therapy intervention in which the therapist provides clients with information about their diagnosis, symptoms, or the method of treatment used. It is more than simply sharing information with the client; it is a therapeutic intervention that delivers information in a structured and sequential manner, facilitating improved decision making, access to resources, and insight for both children and their families.

Thus, psychoeducation includes informing clients and families about various aspects of the condition, including signs and symptoms, course, potential outcomes, and prognosis. In addition, the therapist debunks misconceptions about the condition. Further, the therapist provides information regarding different treatment and medication options, including their risks and benefits (Bhattacharjee et al., 2011). Simply put, information is power, and people turn to information as a way to cope with life situations, as evidenced by the surfeit of popular books on different conditions.

BENEFITS OF PSYCHOEDUCATION WITH PATIENTS WITH NEUROCOGNITIVE IMPAIRMENTS

Explaining the patient's learning and attention challenges in a structured, sequential manner by using psychoeducation techniques can begin to alleviate self-blame and encourage the patient to take a more objective perspective regarding their challenges. Talking openly about learning disorders creates a destigmatized environment in which shameful experiences can be tolerated and discussed. The discussion can then move to deeper work that uncovers the impact of the learning or attentional disability on all facets of the patient's life, including their relationships, self-esteem, and confidence. Psychoeducation helps patients understand that their learning difficulties stem from a neurocognitive etiology and dispels their mistaken ideas that they are lazy, defiant, or stupid. This awareness facilitates acceptance of diverse interventions in the academic and emotional realms as well as improved self-advocacy.

Referencing successful individuals with ADD, LD, or ASD can also emphasize the idea that having learning or attention difficulties does not mean that one cannot succeed or lacks intelligence.

I will now review the literature on the efficacy of psychoeducation with specific disorders.

ADD and Psychoeducation

The positive role of psychoeducation with children and families with ADHD was supported by the majority of studies that were reviewed. In this case, psychoeducation was defined as a specific therapeutic program focusing on didactic communication to patients and families about the condition as well as relevant coping skills (Montoya et al., 2011). For example, a blind, randomized controlled trial of 81 children and adolescents with ADHD found that psychoeducation improved attention and reduced stress and family conflict (Ferrin et al., 2014). Likewise, numerous critical reviews of studies examining psychoeducational approaches to ADHD found that providing educational information increased both knowledge and positive attitudes and behaviors among parents and children (Ferrin e.t al, 2020; Nussey et al., 2013). The following case example illustrates the benefits of psychoeducation with children with ADHD.

Michael, a bright, 15-year-old high school student at a highly competitive school, entered treatment subsequent to experiencing significant anxiety caused by poor performance. He described difficulty doing his work, submitting assignments, and studying for tests. This pattern began in elementary school, but he was able to "get by" with his intelligence and excellent memory. However, the demands of this rigorous school were overwhelming for him, and he failed his math class. A neuropsychological evaluation revealed attention deficit disorder and relatively weaker visual-spatial skills. Michael was enthusiastic about the results as they made sense to him and explained his challenges, particularly in math. The psychoeducation component of this intervention focused on explaining the impact of his attention challenges and poor visual-spatial skills on his ability to perform academically. The first few months of the treatment centered around helping Michael come up with specific strategies to address his attention challenges and math deficits, that is, problem solving. Interventions included working with an organizational coach, figuring out the best place to work at home, and establishing accountability. In addition, I recommended organizing the math problems so there were one or two per page, using larger graph paper, and highlighting and underlining signs and numbers so he could complete his work more efficiently.

Learning Disorders and Psychoeducation

Psychoeducation is commonly used to help parents and children understand their learning disorders, resulting in decreased parental stress and increased understanding of the child's behavior (Brock et al., 2001). In addition, participation in psychoeducation groups facilitated transition planning for students with learning disorders (Milsom et al., 2004). This group model increased disability self-awareness and promoted self-advocacy skills. Thus, acquiring information about the specific learning disability is essential for both the child and the parent to feel more comfortable with the diagnosis and more readily access treatment options. A case example of working with a child with dyslexia highlights the benefits of this approach.

> Adam presented as a bright, engaging 8-year-old boy at a competitive school who was struggling with reading and attention difficulties. Upon receiving a diagnosis of dyslexia and discussing it extensively with the therapist, he happily announced his diagnosis to his class. He created a signup sheet for his peers to ask him questions about his diagnosis. When confronted with a word problem in math, he stated, "I have dyslexia, so I may need help with reading the problem." He then proceeded to do the problem independently and confidently. Receiving the diagnosis and understanding his problems helped him advocate for himself successfully.

Psychoeducation is equally valuable to the parent of a child with learning disabilities. The parent's anxiety about the child's future is often triggered and his or her wishes regarding the child may make it difficult to accept the diagnosis. As the parents are able to voice their concerns and get information about the disorder, they can better understand their children's challenges.

> A highly successful lawyer brought in her 4-year-old daughter, Anna for testing due to concern with the child's language development. In the intake, the mother cried as she described her wish for her daughter to succeed academically and to attend a competitive private school. During an extended consultation period, the mother was able to accept the diagnosis of auditory processing disorder (APD) and to support realistic potential placements where her daughter would be more likely to flourish academically.

Autistic Spectrum Disorder (ASD) and Psychoeducation

Patients with ASD often require psychoeducation as they do not understand their own symptoms. In fact, psychoeducation about ASD is one of the guidelines of good post-diagnostic care (Johnson et al., 2007; Lipinski et al., 2021). Similarly, evaluation of a group psychoeducation program for young people with ASD raised awareness of the disorder and facilitated insight (Gordon et al., 2014). Further studies confirmed the effectiveness of psychoeducation for older adolescents, facilitating a sense of empowerment (Backman et al., 2018). Additionally, parents of children with ASD require significant psychoeducation as ASD symptoms can be easily misunderstood. For example, their children's rigidity can be seen as oppositionist, their responses to sensory overload can be construed as being "bratty" and their anxiety can be masked by defensiveness. In studies of psychoeducational intervention models, parent psychoeducation regarding ASD was shown to decrease parenting stress and improve knowledge about ASD (Patra et al. 2015; Hemdi & Daley, 2017; Magana et al., 2017). The following case example illustrates the benefits of parental understanding of the diagnosis.

A mother was concerned about her son's consistent reluctance to try new foods and activities and to tolerate breaks in routine. The test results indicated that her son met diagnostic criteria for autistic spectrum disorder (ASD). He approached the world with an overly rigid approach to situations, concrete understanding of language, and poor ability to negotiate change. When I explained the etiology of his refusal to try new activities, the mother was able to work more effectively with her son to prepare him for change and to regulate her reactions when he had difficulty with transitions. Knowing that her son had neurocognitive impairments helped her move away from feeling that he was simply a "brat." She was able to empathize with him and intervene more effectively when he was having trouble.

Psychoeducation is conducted in tandem with insight-oriented work to uncover the etiology of low self-esteem and to help the patient cope with feelings of frustration and shame that are related to both past experiences and current life choices. In my own work, I tackle many of these issues from a psychodynamic framework as this approach prioritizes the impact of early childhood experiences on personality development. As noted above, psychoeducation continues throughout the treatment as awareness of the impact of the disability ebbs and flows depending on the life stressors and the internal preoccupations of the patient. I will now discuss the use of a psychodynamic approach with patients with neurocognitive challenges.

PSYCHOTHERAPY INTERVENTIONS

Psychodynamic Approach

Once the patient has accepted that he or she has an LD and/or ADD, is fairly well informed about their specific challenges, and has begun to explore different strategies and aids to compensate for these issues, the insight-oriented piece of the treatment can move to the foreground. Insight is always a piece of the work, as simply discussing the disorders can be both challenging to and ameliorative of self-esteem. However, once the emphasis on the practical and logistical pieces recedes, the patient's feelings about their challenges and the emotional impact they have had come into sharper focus. At this juncture, the therapist can facilitate the patient's delving into early memories of the disorder along with painful experiences of disapproval and disappointment, ultimately helping them rebuild their confidence.

Psychodynamic or psychoanalytically-informed treatment is an excellent vehicle for these tasks. Some of the hallmarks of psychodynamic treatment include focus upon the (1) unconscious nature of many patients' motivations and emotions, (2) effects of childhood experiences on adult emotional life, (3) development and centrality of the perception of self and others, and (4) ways the patients' learned ways of perceiving self and others plays out in the therapeutic relationship (i.e., transference and countertransference). This latter feature will be dealt with in a later chapter. Historically, psychoanalytic/psychodynamic therapists have shied away from treating patients with neurocognitive impairments; however there has been a significant shift in recent decades to include these patients in psychoanalytically informed treatment (Gensler, 1993; Sinason, 2002; Shedler, 2010; Bucholtz, 1987). Psychodynamic treatment can help patients better understand the etiology of their psychiatric symptoms and improve self-esteem, self-confidence, and self-regulation (Shedler, 2010; Huprich, 2009). As patients with neurocognitive impairments have generally experienced significant stress and disruptions in their interpersonal relationships, both as children and as adults, psychodynamic treatment can help them understand these ruptures and subsequently improve social and emotional functioning. I will not go into the full complexities of psychoanalytic work here as these are beyond the scope of this book. Rather I will discuss in a limited way how to apply psychodynamic principles to the treatment of patients with neurocognitive challenges.

One of the most devastating experiences when struggling with learning/attention deficits is the repeated experiences of failure that can set the stage for low self-esteem, anxiety, and depression. Now, such shameful experiences of failure are experienced by different individuals to different degrees and no two patients are alike. Nonetheless, it has been a powerful and persistent theme in my work with patients with neurocognitive challenges.

Understanding, sympathizing with, tolerating, and metabolizing these feelings are among the most crucial tasks a therapist, parent, tutor, or anyone else who works with these children must move toward (Orenstein., 2000). In adult treatment, finding and chipping away at these painful self-perceptions and experiences of rejection is essential to helping the patient gain confidence and improve self-esteem.

When patients tell me they feel stupid or like a fraud, they are relating feelings of embarrassment associated with their learning issues. I often ask my patients what it means to them to sit in a classroom and not be able to conform to the expectations of their teachers and their peers. I ask, "How did it feel being unable to perform?" In doing so, I am addressing possibly hidden or obscured feelings of shame head on.

Discussion of these shameful experiences reduces the shame by helping patients feel less alone with their feelings and by helping them feel compassionate about their struggles, rather than judgmental. The therapist can accomplish this by directly empathizing with the patient's perspective, modeling compassion and a nonjudgmental approach, and pointing out the toxic cycle that the shame has produced. By confronting their feelings, patients can begin to let go of some of the negative self-concepts and better understand their challenges. I encourage my patients to understand that they felt bewildered, frustrated, overwhelmed, and inadequate due to their neurocognitive issues. Once they can more fully understand and empathize with their own experiences, they can better tolerate techniques to improve their actual performance. The challenges of helping the patient shift perspectives and reframe the learning disability in a more constructive fashion comes up with all my patients who exhibit these disorders. They tend to cling tenaciously to the narrative that they are stupid or lazy, and these ideas get brought back into the treatment for years.

In addition, professional and/or academic setbacks can revive these ideas and experiences. I then need to remind the patients about the psychoeducation perspective and delve deeper into the pain and trauma related to the disorder.

I will now address specific implications of each disorder when treating patients psychodynamically.

Attention Deficit Disorder and Psychodynamic Therapy

Psychodynamic therapy is indicated for patients with ADD as their poor impulse control and compromised organization skills often lead to intense conflict with parents, teachers, peers, bosses, and colleagues. The constant feedback about their deficits from others leads to feelings of shame and maladaptive coping strategies. Psychodynamic intervention helps facilitate self-awareness, improves impulse control, and ameliorates these potent feelings of shame. Despite these advantages, the psychodynamic literature on ADD is sparse, although psychodynamic therapy has been shown to be effective with children with ADHD in research and clinical studies (Barzegary & Zamini, 2011; Conway, 2017; Salmonsson, 2006). Likewise, Carney (2002) described treating an adult patient using attachment theory to improve affect regulation. The power of words in the therapeutic situation was highlighted, as ADHD children can interpret language concretely and the therapist needs to be mindful of this challenge and choose their words carefully (Salmonsson, 2008). I will now provide a case example to illustrate the integration of psychoeducation, accommodations, and psychodynamic therapy in the treatment of individuals with attention deficit disorder.

> Joe, a young adult who was diagnosed with ADD as a child, initially entered treatment following a neuropsychological evaluation that revealed that he was a highly intelligent, capable, and well-related young man with significant attentional deficits. One coping mechanism that he used throughout school was to entertain his peers and use his high energy level to socialize and participate in class. However, due to his difficulty focusing, he invariably fell short when it came to grades and assignments. His mother was very critical about his poor grades, and this further contributed to his sense of inadequacy and humiliation. As a college student, he struggled with depression and poor motivation. In treatment, I encouraged him to take medicine, work with an academic support tutor, and understand how his ADD had impacted his ability to have "passion" and motivation. He continued to express that he did not feel intrinsically motivated and engaged in his work. He struggled with profound feelings of depression and continued to withdraw interpersonally as well as academically. As we discussed these feelings, memories surfaced of being berated by his mother for poor work as well as getting in trouble in class for his impulsivity. He uncovered that his response to these experiences was to withdraw from the academic arena and shift his attention into socializing and smoking marijuana. After these discussions, he was then able to take more responsibility for his work and begin to work more independently. Recently, he discussed his concerns about being successful professionally and how to incorporate his learning style and high level of energy into a work environment.

This case highlights the role of shame when individuals underperform and how they may defend against this shame by avoiding tasks. This defense further exacerbates the problem of poor performance as family members, teachers, bosses, and friends may react with frustration and feel put off when the person cannot take initiative or exert effort academically or professionally in therapy, exploring the etiology for the poor performance and the shame surrounding it can increase awareness of the motivation behind the maladaptive coping mechanisms. Ultimately this can enhance patients' willingness to take charge of their own behavior, which then fosters success across multiple important domains. Shame is only one of the feelings that can arise when individuals perform poorly due to their neurocognitive challenges. People can also feel angry, frustrated, depressed, and avoidant. However, in my experience, shame is a particularly potent and difficult to express feeling that needs to be addressed in treatment.

Learning Disorders and Psychodynamic Therapy

As mentioned above, in the past, psychoanalysis has discouraged treatment for individuals with learning disorders. However, in more recent decades, there is increased documentation of the efficacy of insight-oriented therapy to help patients accept their learning disabilities, come up with realistic strategies to cope with their lives, and resolve the stress and trauma caused by the learning challenges (Gensler, 1993; Rothstein & Glenn, 1999). Likewise, Palombo (2001) proposed a detailed theoretical and clinical approach to difficulties with self-regulation and identity among children with learning disorders. Further, attachment research and advances in our understanding of early infant-mother interactions have been used successfully to treat individuals with learning disorders (Erdheim & Niedecken, 1998; Sinason, 2002; Hollins & Sinason, 2000). I will now present two case examples of psychodynamic work with patients with learning disorders.

One of my patients with a long-standing history of a nonverbal LD and good insight into her internal conflicts, referred to her perfectionist and self-critical sense as the "tyrant." The "tyrant" was a demeaning and harsh self-state where she did not feel she could have friends or succeed in school. In discussing her social and performance anxiety, I encouraged her to talk back to the "tyrant" and protect the little girl who had been so cruelly shunned and rejected. Over time, she joined a club at college, began to socialize and, although the "tyrant" still spoke up from time to time, she was much better able to dismiss these thoughts and continue working towards her goal of having a satisfying social life.

In another case, Susan, a young adult with multiple learning and attention challenges as well as psychiatric issues, often referred to herself as "SPED" (special education) in a harsh and derogatory manner. Recently, she was accepted into a prestigious graduate program and began discussing with me her intention to preview the curriculum and figure out what accommodations and support she would need in order to succeed. As we were discussing her distress regarding not being able to access the curriculum prior to starting classes, she became very agitated, triggering an escalating spiral of catastrophic thoughts. She said that she had initially been waitlisted for the program and then got accepted off the waitlist. This meant that she has a black mark against her, is once again "SPED," and will require special help. Therefore, the program director will think negatively about her, and she will not be able to succeed. We discussed how her early education struggles and her feeling different from her peers has impacted her current perceptions about her graduate program. We devised a plan for support and accommodations with which she felt comfortable and reinforced that we would need to continue discussing her feelings, as being back in school would likely be triggering for her.

Autism Spectrum Disorder and Psychodynamic Therapy

Individuals with autism spectrum disorder (ASD) typically seek out treatment to address feelings of depression and anxiety. In addition, they often present with obsessive compulsive symptoms and impairments in social communication and relationships (Lipinski et al., 2018; Koenig & Levine, 2012). Alvarez (1992) writes extensively about treatment with autistic children utilizing psychoanalytic techniques; she focuses on the use of play and the therapist's ability to make sense of the patient's world. Despite interest and need for treatment, many individuals with ASD have difficulty accessing treatment as many therapists are reluctant to treat them due to misconceptions about the disorder (Lipinski et al., 2022.) Therapists may assume that patients with ASD are too concrete to benefit from insight-oriented therapy. In addition, as individuals with ASD express emotions and relate to people in an atypical manner, these interpersonal and emotional deficits may seem like challenges to treatment. However, individuals with ASD are receptive to treatment despite these obstacles and can benefit greatly from insight, awareness, and the therapeutic relationship.

Alex, a young adult with a self-diagnosis of ASD, came into treatment due to concerns about overwhelming anxiety, chronic depression, and a host of other symptoms that he attributed to ASD—including hypersensitivity to sensory stimuli, such as noise, light, and social interactions. He also complained of "burn out," that is, low energy, difficulty accomplishing tasks, and poor focus. Treatment initially centered on helping him express distress regarding varied stressful life events, including having become mentally ill in high school. He had been high functioning through the middle of eighth grade, then had an apparent breakdown that required partial hospitalization and special school placement in high school. Prior to this, he had been a competitive athlete but after his breakdown, he was no longer able to compete athletically, which was extremely distressing for him. As we worked through his past trauma, we began to focus on helping Alex regulate his responses and become more productive academically. He developed self-regulation tools, such as taking a break as needed, regulating his environment, and engaging in hobbies. After a year in therapy, he graduated from high school and enrolled in college by taking part-time classes. Recently, he spoke poignantly about not being able to go on a class trip due to overwhelming anxiety and sensitivity to stimuli. We discussed alternate ways to participate in the class and to feel proud of his progress in attending the class at all.

Although psychodynamic treatments offer many benefits in terms of working through the long-lasting effects of painful past experiences, treatment for patients with neurocognitive challenges typically requires a wider array of techniques.

Multi-Modal Approaches

In general, psychotherapy should be provided in a nuanced manner, specifically tailored to the patient and often incorporating multiple approaches. Many patients demonstrate significant overlap between executive functioning disorder, attention deficit disorder, and other learning disorders. In addition, anxiety and depression are common, given the myriad of academic and social challenges. Interventions should therefore be tailored to account for the overlap between these deficits. Use of multiple modalities, such as CBT, DBT, play and insight-oriented therapy, is often necessary given the diverse symptoms and complex challenges. For example, CBT can reduce anxiety, curb intrusive thoughts, and reduce impulsivity. DBT can improve coping skills, enhance interpersonal skills, and improve flexibility and problem solving. Play therapy as a means of insight-oriented work for children can help children recognize and communicate their emotions and conflicts and in so doing improve self-esteem, reduce shame, improve confidence, and enhance one's ability to connect with peers and adults in a substantive manner. CBT and DBT are time-limited interventions that utilize a manual-based approach. In contrast, play therapy and insight-oriented therapy utilize an open-ended approach in terms of time, structure, and format; the focus is on developing a relationship with children and helping them work through their conflicts and challenges either by verbal discussion or symbolically processing them via imaginative play or board games. Play therapy is more creative and spontaneous than the manual-based therapies and intervenes in a more global fashion regarding relationships, self-esteem, and overall social-emotional functioning.

Cognitive Behavior Therapy

Cognitive Behavior Therapy (CBT) is a psycho-social intervention that teaches coping skills and focuses on how your thoughts, beliefs and attitudes affect your feelings and behaviors. It is one of the most widely used therapeutic interventions with children and adults with attention deficit disorders as it targets specific symptoms and behaviors and is well suited for skills training (Braswell & Bloomquist, 1991; Jensen et al. 2016). Both research and clinical studies have documented its efficacy in improving impulse control, reducing aggression, and reducing symptoms of inattention (Miranda & Presentacion, 2000). As children with learning disorders often have behavioral problems, behavior management techniques have been commonly used to help manage symptoms related to poor frustration tolerance and anxiety. Dagnan et al. (2016) discussed the use of CBT to alleviate emotional distress and improve self-management.

Kopelman-Rubin (2012) describes a promising intervention with adolescents diagnosed with learning disorders based on an interpersonal model for treating depressed adolescents (Mufson et al., 1994). The intervention includes the adolescent, parent and school staff and focuses upon improving interpersonal skills, promoting self-awareness, and facilitating increased support for the adolescent from parents and the school.

Cognitive behavior therapy can also be applicable to some of the specific symptoms presented by individuals with ASD. As it is skill-driven, the treatment can improve communication and social skills (Beebe & Risi, 2003). Cognitive behavioral treatment programs consist of breaking down the behavior into discrete units, targeting each skill in a hierarchical manner and scaffolding the patient to help them demonstrate the expected behaviors. For example, they can work on improving eye contact, engaging in conversation, and, through graduated and repeated exposure, desensitizing to social situations to reduce anxiety. A review of CBT programs targeting anxiety, disruptive behavior, and core autism symptoms for children with autism indicated that CBT is possibly effective but called for more research (Danial & Wood, 2013). However, a meta-analysis of randomized, controlled trials of CBT in children and adolescents with high functioning autism supported its efficacy in reducing anxiety (Sukhodolsky et al., 2013).

Cognitive behavioral therapy has also shown to improve social skill deficits in teens with high functioning autism (White et al., 2010). As social communication deficits are one of the hallmarks of ASD, social skills training is a valuable intervention. There is increasing evidence that comprehensive social skills training, using CBT, in conjunction with art and insight-oriented therapy can improve social skills in these patients (Epp, 2008; McConachie, 2013).

Group Therapy

Group therapy is an excellent adjunctive treatment that, along with medication, individual therapy, and parent training, can improve social and emotional functioning in patients with neurocognitive challenges (Waxmonsky et al., 2012). Group therapy is a powerful tool to reduce stigma and isolation as it introduces patients to other people with similar difficulties. In addition, it offers opportunities to improve social skills, enhance attention to interpersonal nuances and reduce social anxiety. The group format provides a unique therapeutic experience as patients obtain immediate feedback from peers, are able to learn from others' experiences and practice socializing with peers in a structured and supportive environment.

Social skills training in a group format is a valuable adjunctive treatment for children with learning disorders as their neurocognitive challenges often lead to interpersonal difficulties (as discussed in Chapter 3). Nonetheless, although it can bring about real-life opportunities to strengthen social competence, group therapy alone is not always sufficient to improve peer relations (Ogilvy, 1994; Zaragoza et al., 1991). Mishna et al. (1994) advocated for group therapy in combination with individual therapy to improve social adjustment with children with learning disabilities. Likewise, Waxmonsky et al. (2012) has documented the efficacy of group therapy combined with parent training for children with ADHD.

For clients with language-based learning disorders, the group provides necessary practice in engaging in banter, initiating, and sustaining conversations, and role playing how to express their feelings and advocate for themselves with family members, teachers, and friends. For clients with visual-spatial learning disorders, the group affords them the opportunity to attend to social nuances, pick up on social cues and analyze social situations in a safe environment. Individuals with attention deficit disorder learn how to improve impulse control, reduce disruptive behavior, such as interruptions, and improve attending to others in conversations. Lastly, clients with ASD greatly benefit from a social outlet where they can practice social interactions and improve communication skills.

I run a clinical group of college-aged adults who present with diverse learning, attention, and psychiatric challenges. Issues related to obtaining academic accommodations, resolving conflict with parents, reaching out to friends, and understanding the impact of their learning issues are all regularly discussed. I try to structure my interventions around this shared experience, and often introduce them by saying, for example, "All of us in this room have experienced the frustration of trying to explain our learning struggles to family members." Statements like these help the group members relate to one another. They facilitate an atmosphere of mutual understanding while inviting the exploration of each patient's own specific experiences and emotions—such as feeling stupid, misunderstood, frustrated, and ashamed. An excerpt of a group session illustrates these themes:

> One session began with a student reaching out for support from the group regarding her difficulty completing assignments in a timely manner and her reluctance to advocate for extended time on deadlines. Other patients chimed in and expressed strategies for obtaining necessary services as well as the gamut of mixed emotions accompanying obtaining support. They discussed feeling angry that they are set apart from their peers and the fantasy that everyone else is able to complete their work better than they can. There is also both a sense of relief and guilt that they are receiving special treatment. The feelings of guilt and shame were very powerful and echoed by all the group members. As we discussed their past experiences with teachers, parents, and peers, group members teared up and supported one another. At the end of the group, the members brainstormed strategies on how to obtain extended time and discussed how facing their learning issues and advocating for accommodations enabled them to flourish academically.

Parent Guidance

Guidance for parents is a crucial part of the treatment for children and adolescents with learning and attentional disorders. As children with neurocognitive challenges present significant parenting challenges, parent training is an excellent adjunctive treatment to reduce stress and conflict at home. Parents often feel at a loss in how best to help their children and can also benefit from support in dealing with the difficult emotions that arise when raising a child with special learning needs. Parent training was shown to be an effective behavioral intervention in a double-blind, placebo-controlled study (Horn et al., 1991). In children with ASD, parent training programs have been shown to improve communication, reduce autistic symptoms in children, and reduce parent-child conflict (Matson et al., 2009; Bearss et al., 2015; Postorino et al., 2017). Similarly, self-compassion training was found to be an effective treatment with parents with children with learning disorders (Vanestanagh, 2020).

A number of interventions have been designed to work with parents. Parent-Child Interaction Therapy (PCIT) seems to be a promising intervention, particularly with young children with ADHD (Wagner & McNeil, 2007). This therapy is a structured behavioral program that coaches parents how to set limits and help their children conform to behavioral expectations. The parents work with the children with the guidance of the therapist in the office environment. A randomized, controlled trial of PCIT with children with ADD demonstrated a significant decrease in child behavior and attention problems, parental stress and an increase in positive parenting practices (Leung et al., 2016).

MODIFICATIONS OF THERAPEUTIC STYLES

In addition to integrating multiple therapeutic modalities, work with children and adults with neurocognitive challenges often requires modification of standard therapeutic techniques. For example, I frequently modify my communication style when working with patients with different disorders, utilize a hand-on approach to help scaffold academic and other tasks for patients, and extend the therapy beyond the patient and family to incorporate a team approach with other professionals.

Therapeutic Styles for Specific Disorders

Understanding the impact of diverse learning styles in treatment helps the therapist adjust his/her expectations and use different techniques to work with the patient. I employ specific strategies in the treatment to accommodate diverse learning styles. For example, I exaggerate my facial expressions to convey feelings when working with individuals with nonverbal learning disorders. I will convey insight and suggestions in a concrete, highly structured manner for individuals with language-based learning disabilities to ensure that they assimilate the information in an effective manner. I will text patients between sessions to remind them of their goals or tasks to accommodate those patients with ADD who have difficulty remembering their commitments. I am mindful that my patients with ASD can easily misperceive social situations and act as a reality check for them as they recount their social challenges.

Hands On Approach

Patients with LD, ADD, and ASD often require more direct support, particularly regarding task-completion, due to their executive functioning deficits. I often write texts or send emails with the patient, both to help them get organized and to reduce the anxiety associated with the task. If I do not help them with their work directly, I often suggest a resource such as a tutor or executive functioning coach who can offer the support and scaffolding that they require. Scaffolding is a technique of helping students master complex problems by breaking down the task into a sequence of manageable chunks.

Sitting with patients as they complete their work allows me to experience their anxiety directly and offer support and scaffolding as they begin to negotiate working independently. The therapist can provide practical coaching in real time to help patients tackle challenging and daunting tasks (Sorscher, 2019). For example, we may draw up a schedule helping them organize test preparation and assignment completion, write an essay together, or use the time to read a text together. Gensler (personal communication, March 18, 2021) uses the online format (necessitated during the pandemic) to join the child in his or her world. He encourages child patients to share the screen and show him their homework. They will also play video games together, watch movies, or take a tour of the children's rooms. Rolling up your sleeves with the child, letting him or her know you are available to join in real time, and supporting his or her modes of self-expression improves attention and rapport in therapy, as well as the child's academic and social skills. While patients may need support to get started on specific tasks, successive experiences of mastery will help them move to greater levels of independence.

Advocacy and Team Approach

Effective intervention includes figuring out a personalized plan for each patient that keeps both their neurocognitive and psychiatric needs in mind. These strategies may include having the patients work with different professionals, that is, a tutor, speech therapist, executive functioning coach, or personal assistant. To improve coordination of the team of professionals that is often assembled to support the patient, the therapist can be in touch with other providers on a regular basis. I spearhead a team approach to establish team meetings, initiate clinical communication, prevent splitting and advocate for the patient with parents, teachers, tutors, and other specialists. Explaining the child's needs and the etiology of his or her behaviors helps the people on the "front line" manage their expectations of the child, be more helpful to the child and prevent burn out.

I recently tested a bright, verbal ninth grader who had a history of spending hours studying for math tests, but still received poor grades. Testing revealed he was an auditory learner who would get overwhelmed with visual information and instead felt most comfortable, and ultimately successful, when words were used to explain math concepts. He felt lost and confused because, like most math educators, his teacher used visual cues—in this case, numbers—to explain concepts. Once I shared his learning style with his parents and tutor, they began putting math concepts into words and finding mnemonics for the math operations he needed to perform. For example, before starting an assignment, he developed a written checklist of the steps required to complete algebra problems. He began writing his notes and procedures in words instead of numbers and "talking his assignments out," essentially, discussing his assignments with his parents and tutor and reviewing his notes aloud. Once these strategies were implemented, his grades improved.

This story of success is not unique to this student. When adults understand the child's learning style, they can create study habits to build confidence and accomplishment.

The team approach is especially useful when the child receives multiple services and requires a nuanced understanding of their complex needs.

For example, I worked with John, a third grader with ADD which impacted his social/emotional and academic functioning. John received speech/language, OT and individual and group therapy. Team meetings to coordinate services were held quarterly with parents and teachers. Goals for behavior and expectations were discussed and reviewed. Explaining the interface between sensory issues and disruptive behavior was essential to help the parents and teachers modify their expectations of John. I also helped the team come up with strategies to help John conform to rules and routines at school, such as not wearing his sunglasses, taking off his hat and reducing playing with objects on his desk. Likewise, John was easily distracted by peers, so his seat was moved to a quieter area.

In sum, individuals with neurocognitive challenges benefit from an integrated intervention approach that is tailored to their specific disorder. This approach combines psychoeducation, problem-solving strategies and insight-oriented treatment to facilitate insight, improve self-esteem, and address the social/emotional impact of their areas of deficit. Group therapy is a very useful adjunctive treatment to ameliorate distress, combat social isolation and improve social/emotional functioning. Parent training has also been identified as an essential adjunctive treatment to reduce family stress and improve relationships.

Chapter Seven

Transference/Countertransference Issues in the Assessment and Treatment of Individuals with Neurocognitive Challenges

A cornerstone of psychodynamic therapy is the consideration of transference/countertransference issues as central to the therapy. Transference occurs when patients transfer their feelings about someone else onto the therapist. Typically, this refers to feelings toward earlier attachment figures encapsulated in early childhood schemas. Countertransference occurs when the therapist transfers his or her feelings onto the patient. This may refer to deep-seated interpersonal representations but also daily emotional reactions. It can also reflect the therapist's reaction to the patient's transference. Both transference and countertransference can be useful in the therapeutic relationship because they illustrate the patient's issues and bring them to life in the consulting room. It is important to consider the common transference/countertransference reactions in the treatment of patients with neurocognitive challenges as these dynamics often play a critical role in the therapy and successful management of such patterns is often crucial to the treatment. Recognizing how patients experience and relate to the therapist gives us a mirror into their self-perception and of how they relate to others. Therapists' countertransference offers another valuable lens with which to appreciate patients' impact on those around them and to allow the therapist to gain an experience-near appreciation of the patients' emotional life. Working through these issues helps patients improve their interpersonal relationships and enhance insight. As these dynamics come into play in the testing as well as the therapy, I will discuss themes of transference/countertransference that arise in assessment as well as therapy with patients with neurocognitive challenges.

Understanding the patient's response to having a learning disability is crucial for appreciating the underpinnings of the transference, as such feelings will color their responses to the therapist. As noted in earlier chapters, having a learning/attention disorder leaves one vulnerable to intense feelings of shame, guilt, resentment, frustration, low self-esteem, anxiety, and depression—all of which are likely to emerge in the transference/countertransference. In order to cope with these painful feelings, patients with learning disorders often hide their deficits. They may adamantly deny their challenges, avoid any references to their disabilities, and become oppositional and negativistic when confronted with tasks that are challenging for them. They may devalue the task, the therapist, and anyone else related to the task—such as teachers or bosses. These responses will be reenacted in the treatment and require careful consideration. Treatment with individuals with autism spectrum disorder may also encompass these themes and responses. In addition, the transference that they develop is marked by their difficulty accessing emotions and engaging in interpersonal relationships.

COMMON TRANSFERENCE REACTIONS OF PATIENTS

Addressing neurocognitive deficits in therapy will typically force patients to expose something that they may have tried to hide for most of their life, triggering significant shame and frustration. As people tend to naturally shy away from feelings of humiliation, it is very difficult for patients with neurocognitive deficits to access, understand, and tolerate those feelings. The patient may become evasive, resist the therapist's exploration, and leave the therapist in the dark. When the deficit is revealed, the patient may feel exposed, defensive, and resentful—and may even become aggressive. He or she may also avoid therapy in an attempt to avoid the pain associated with confronting these challenges.

In the patient's mind, the therapist comes to represent the authority figures involved with childhood learning experiences, such as teachers or parents. How patients experienced these figures in the context of their learning challenges greatly informs the transference. I have found that patients often treat me the way they have been treated, that is, critically, and dismissively. My patients often report feelings of shame when recounting instances during which they were unable to understand a teacher's lecture, keep up with peers, or succeed academically and/or socially. When parents and teachers respond to these shortcomings with disappointment, the child may either internalize these painful feelings or wield their anger against the adult as a way of distancing themselves from pain. A similar situation can arise in therapy: the therapist may be a disappointing figure to the patient or seen as disappointed *in* the patient. The therapist can disappoint patients by misunderstanding their feelings, by miscommunicating an interpretation, or by providing them with too little or too much information. These patient-therapist impasses need to be understood against the backdrop of the patient's learning difficulties, as they are replications of past situations where the patient did not understand information or could not communicate his or her ideas effectively and felt judged because of it.

Patients may also become very agitated and aggressive if they feel the therapist is exposing or humiliating them by discussing their learning challenges. The patient may feel annoyed at the therapist's perceived intrusiveness, but concurrently grateful to the therapist for their support with tasks. They may feel frustrated that the therapist is not helpful enough or angry if they feel pressure from the therapist to take on tasks that make them anxious. They may also be concerned about disappointing the therapist if they are unable to complete tasks successfully or advocate for themselves in a school or work setting. In response to suggestions for accommodations, patients may feel defensive and unfairly singled out. They may feel unworthy of and resistant to intervention as if they are receiving special privileges or cheating. Providing clients with tools they can employ on their own can be seen as supportive and loving but also as infantilizing. Thus, by providing the very help that the patient needs, the therapist can elicit an angry, defensive, and resistant response. Additionally, patients diagnosed with specific neurocognitive challenges tend to present specific types of transference reactions and are apt to provoke distinct countertransference responses.

Attention Deficit Disorder

Patients with ADD may conduct themselves in the session in a chaotic and disorganized manner. For example, they may often come late, miss sessions, ask to change the time of their regular session frequently and have difficulty sitting still or maintaining focus throughout the session. In addition, they may communicate in a tangential manner, get easily distracted and have difficulty attending to what the therapist is communicating. They may perceive the therapist as rigid and demanding as they have trouble conforming to the therapeutic frame. These challenges should not be interpreted as resistance, defensiveness, or avoidance as they are neurocognitive in etiology. The therapist can work with the patients on coming up with systems and strategies to facilitate improved compliance with both the framework of the sessions, that is, the time, and the content of the sessions, that is, the conversations. For example, I always text my patients with ADD with a reminder about their sessions and I encourage them to take notes during the session if they have trouble remembering our discussions. A case example illustrates these points.

Alex, a highly verbal young adult with ADD, frequently arrived late for his sessions. When I expressed interest in his routine and how he organized his schedule, he recounted a highly disorganized approach to his life. He often stayed at work late and then invariably would wake up late, miss important meetings, and incur disappointment from his colleagues. I encouraged Alex to commit to a schedule that allowed him to leave work on time and gave him more time for leisure pursuits. As Alex worked on these habits, I noticed that his punctuality improved in therapy.

Psychodynamic treatment offers the opportunity for the child to feel understood as compared with other treatment models that focus on external behaviors and may perpetuate the child's sense of being criticized. (Cione et al., 2011; Jones, 2002). Gilmore (2000) noted that ADHD children often present with competitive and envious feelings that are managed with defenses such as identification with the aggressor (Gilmore, 2000); thus, psychodynamic, transference-oriented treatment is well suited to detect and work to modify these defenses as they are enacted in the transference. Gensler (2011) thoughtfully explored the interplay between the patients' attention difficulties and its impact on the therapist's ability to attend to the patients. As patients begin to be able to pay better attention to themselves and their world, the therapist was able to attend more effectively to the patients and particularly notice their different self-states.

When working with adults with neurocognitive deficits, the psychoanalytic model of understanding transferences also extends to understanding transferential feelings towards family members, bosses, and peers. Discussing these experiences in the context of the patient's neurocognitive deficits can be very illuminating and facilitate insight and improved interpersonal relationships. The following case history illustrates this point.

Steve, a young man, presented to therapy complaining of anxiety. In working with him, however, it became clear that he had undiagnosed learning issues. Despite being bright and verbal, he struggled to complete his homework, study for tests, and focus on class. He was diagnosed with ADD in third grade and was given medication, which he resented—and because of which he felt stigmatized. As a young adult, he would still have angry blowups with his mother during which he would accuse her of being "stupid" and having "brain damage." As we discussed these outbursts, he was able to connect his rage at his mother to his own fears of being criticized and rejected for his poor academic performance, of his being called stupid or brain damaged himself.

Learning Disorders

Palombo (2001) outlines a treatment approach with children and adolescents with learning disorders that focuses on the therapeutic process as open-ended, with "complementary" moments where the transference and countertransference are addressed. As learning disorders often lead to difficulty establishing a secure sense of self and compromise the ability to initiate and sustain interpersonal relationships, the treatment is often marked by "disjunctive" moments, that is, moments where the child feels misunderstood by the therapist or the therapist misunderstands the child. The therapist can intervene effectively in these spheres using the patient's responses (transference) and their own feelings (countertransference) to facilitate development of a more unified sense of self and the ability to interact more effectively. I will now discuss specific learning disorders and their impact on treatment.

Language-Based Learning Disorder

Patients with language-based learning disorders will have difficulty holding up their end of the conversation. Their interactions might be stilted, and they will have trouble expressing their feelings. These patients can feel like they are being put on the spot when asked open ended questions by the therapist and can perceive the therapist as intrusive and insensitive. The therapist can help by providing support and scaffolding during the conversation, giving them choices regarding expression of feelings instead of simply asking open ended questions and allowing for time between responses. A case example illustrates this approach.

> Mark, a shy young adult, demonstrated significant language issues that prevented him from expressing his ideas. He would often get flustered when talking and exclaim, "Words!" as a way to express his frustration about his difficulty talking. I used scaffolding techniques, such as encouraging him to take his time and role-playing different situations where I gave him the cues to introduce himself and engage in small talk. I also provided prompts such as asking people about their day, commenting on the weather and framing responses to others such as "nice job" and "I agree with you." I offered positive feedback on his insights and ability to engage with his peers. As Mark was able to make productive use of these prompts, his speech became more fluent, he became less frustrated about his speech production and was able to be more productive in therapy.

Nonverbal Learning Disorder

Patients with Nonverbal Learning Disorders can appear flighty and disorganized. They may be tone deaf to interactions and express themselves in an overly blunt, seemingly disrespectful manner. Similarly, they may be oblivious to the space and may inadvertently leave a mess behind them. As time management is a challenge, they may also come late, ask to change the time of the session, and have overall difficulty maintaining a regular schedule. They may view the therapist as unreasonable and rigid when the therapist attempts to discuss any of these issues. The therapist can help by reminding them of the schedule, brainstorming strategies that help them respect the framework and exaggerating his or her own emotional responses to help them understand emotions. Two case examples highlight these points.

Leslie, an anxious young adult with nonverbal learning disorder would often come to session with food that she would eat in a messy fashion. She seemed oblivious to the crumbs she created and would leave the wrapper on the couch. Despite my initial irritation at what felt like her lack of consideration of my space, I was able to discuss these behaviors in a sympathetic manner, letting her know I understood that she did not see the mess, and therefore did not see the need to clean up due to her learning disorder. After initial distress, she was able to associate to having a messy room and messy desk and getting in trouble with her parents and teachers. We discussed her feelings of shame and gradually she began to clean up after herself in the session.

Carl, a young teenage boy with nonverbal learning disorder, often recounted his experiences in a monotone and seemed oblivious to any expressions of boredom or lack of interest in his companions. Although he was a bright boy with engaging areas of interest, he tended to monopolize the conversation and had difficulty engaging in reciprocal conversation. I exaggerated my feelings of boredom by yawning, turning my head away, and sighing. Carl did not immediately pick up on these cues but after I explained these cues to him and encouraged him to observe these responses in others, Carl began to be able to check in with this "audience" (another technique I taught him) and wrap up his stories in a more succinct fashion. This technique of exaggerating emotional responses can be used to good effect in a psychoeducational manner, that is, the clinician explains very clearly to the patient what these cues mean and the reasons why the clinician is employing these cues.

Autism Spectrum Disorder

Patients with autism spectrum disorder may present as withdrawn and poorly related. They may become hyper-fixated on one topic and overwhelm the therapist with an extreme number of details regarding that topic. They are oblivious to social cues and will not register if the therapist is bored. Some of their social deficits are similar to patients with NVLD as described above, however a profound difference is their limited understanding of their own feelings and significant difficulty taking another person's perspective. Thus, they may be bewildered by the therapist's interpretations and have difficulty identifying their emotions. The therapist can help by explaining feelings and interpersonal relationships in a concrete and structured manner. The patient with autism may express a lack of connection and regard for the therapist. Establishing oneself as a stable and secure figure in the patient's life requires time and patience as well as an ability to enter the internal world of the patient. The therapist may feel bored, frustrated, and even rejected by the patient as these patients are so cut off from their own experiences. Entering their world entails engaging them on their terms; being interested in their interests and slowly helping them establish a connection with the therapist. The following case example highlights this topic.

Carl, an adolescent with autism, was obsessed with trains. His main topic of conversation was which trains you could take to get around the city or the country. He became very animated when discussing trains but withdrew and retreated when asked to discuss anything else. We devised a system where he could talk about trains for a certain amount of time but then needed to switch topics and tell me about school, his family or any other topic of interest. Initially, Carl had a great deal of difficulty filling the time that was dedicated to the other topics. However, with support and scaffolding, that is, I presented him with prompts, gave him choices of topics and asked very specific questions, he was able to switch gears and tell me about his classes and weekend activities. It was important for me to maintain interest as he discussed trains although the topic and presentation was often painfully boring for me. This allowed him to feel understood and supported, which facilitated his learning to shift gears to discuss other facets of his life.

UNDERSTANDING AND USING THE COUNTERTRANSFERENCE

The therapist can feel confused and bewildered when presented with the patient's evasive maneuvers or rejection of help. They may also feel disappointed or frustrated by the patient when the patient does not follow through on a goal, rejects an interpretation, or misunderstands the therapist. The patient's deficits may contribute to the therapist's sense of exasperation as patients may come late, not pay their bills on time, or react defensively to feeling exposed. Therapists may also feel resentful of their patients when they feel devalued, dismissed, and attacked by them. Further, feelings of inadequacy may surface as the patients' problems are so intense and seemingly impenetrable to intervention. Countertransferential pitfalls for therapists include defending against their own shame by either withdrawing from, being judgmental of, or retaliating against the patient in reaction to the patient's shame-inducing comments or interactions. Therapists may also feel shame about missing the mark with patients. In addition, it may be tempting to try to analyze the patients' difficulties as if they were a product of unconscious intention instead of recognizing their neurocognitive etiology and helping the patient develop compensatory strategies. Further, empathizing with patients' intense feelings of shame, frustration, and disappointment can feel overwhelming to therapists as they work to serve a containing function.

As these challenges often appear quite intractable, therapists must cultivate patience and understand that it can take a very long time for patients to come to terms with their disorders. Even when patients understand their challenges, new life situations may cause an eruption of the original defenses that had been constructed to cope with their difficulties, and the therapist may need to go back to square one in order to intervene effectively, that is, reiterate the neurocognitive etiology, help patients come up with solutions, commiserate with patients, and help them confront their feelings in order to be able to be productive.

Patients frequently enter treatment either unaware of their learning issues or oblivious to the psychic toll their deficits have caused (Gensler, 1993). Because these experiences are often imbued with acute feelings of shame, discussing these learning issues often feels fraught and dangerous, both to the patient and the therapist. The therapists' ability to acknowledge and understand these moments is therefore imperative to reassuring the patient and alleviating their pain (Stein, 1995). However, the danger is that both the patient and the therapist will recoil and avoid the topic and each other.

Additionally, therapists can unwittingly shame patients by asking them about their goals or work when they might feel ashamed that they have not been able to be productive or accomplish their goals. As such, the therapist must be mindful of the potential to inadvertently shame the patient by dredging up embarrassing feelings when discussing the learning disability, as this can create a feedback loop in which the patient reacts by shaming the therapist. In these cases, each participant then becomes trapped in feelings of inadequacy and humiliation, to which the therapist may also react by withdrawing from or dismissing the patient.

In doing this work, the therapist is often faced with a dilemma—as avoiding the topic can lead to a therapeutic stalemate, but addressing these issues is a minefield due to the explosive nature of deep feelings of shame that get triggered. As it often takes a great deal of time (sometimes years) for the patient to incorporate suggestions and strategies, it is essential that the therapist cultivate patience and flexibility. The therapist must be willing to understand that the suggestions may not work. Offering patients strategies and tools definitely runs the risk that the therapist will feel frustrated and/or rejected when the patients do not use the tools, are dismissive of the help, and appear "stuck" in the mire of their neurocognitive challenges. Additionally, the therapist can be seen as judgmental and pressuring. We can expect expressions of anger against the therapist or others as a defense against the painful feelings and deep frustration the patient has endured as a result of his or her neurocognitive challenges.

I aim to be sensitive, gentle, and collaborative when I make suggestions. In addition, I frequently check in with the patient about how my intervention landed as it can be easy to trigger a negative response given how injurious these experiences are for the patient. The following case examples highlight the impact of shame and frustration in the therapy when discussing tasks that are challenging due to neurocognitive deficits.

Laura, a college student, shared her plans to write her paper over the weekend. When I asked her how it went, she exploded into a diatribe as to how insensitive and "fucked up" the question was: "Don't you know how hard it is for me to get work done?" She felt assaulted and shamed by the question, so she turned around and shamed me for asking an "insensitive" question.

With a different patient, I suggested that she set up a meeting with her teacher to discuss her paper. The next session she came in and tearfully disclosed that she was not able to set up the meeting and was scared that I was disappointed in her. As we explored her feelings, she recounted memories of her father pressuring her to read chapter books and being dismissive of her desires to read picture books. We discussed the importance of her respecting her need to move at her own pace.

This work definitely requires patience as the defenses are very ingrained. As noted above, the therapist can feel frustrated, angry, disappointed, and rejected when the patient responds negatively to suggestions and strategies. This case example illustrates this dilemma.

In another instance, I had an intense countertransferential reaction to the second patient when she was procrastinating on writing a research paper. It was clear to me this research paper posed a huge challenge for her due to her neurocognitive difficulties. I would bring up the paper every week, but she would stonewall me, insisting that she was working on being loving and compassionate with herself and trying not to feel bad about avoiding the paper. Although I appreciated her concern for her self-esteem, I was concerned she would fail the class and put her graduate degree in jeopardy. I became increasingly aggressive in promoting her attention to this project and at one point even said to her "I graduated from graduate school. If you don't graduate, that's up to you." We were then able to discuss my lapse in empathy in the context of her history with her parents and with me. She applied for an incomplete in the class and later finished the paper with one-on-one support from a writing coach.

TRANSFERENCE/COUNTERTRANSFERENCE IN ASSESSMENT

As noted above, transference/countertransference themes come up in testing as well as therapy. Transferentially, the tester may be viewed in many ways: as a judgmental or critical parent, a helpful mentor, a competitor, and more. The parents also may reject the testing information. Conversely, they may too readily agree with the tester's perspective. They may feel envious of the tester's information about the child. They may feel judged by the tester. They may also feel dependent on the tester for help and support. For example, they may ask the tester how to help them navigate daily life with the child, advocate for the child at school and make important decisions about the child, including educational and treatment options.

Children also experience significant transferential feelings during testing. The tester is in a position of power, and thus stimulates anxiety, distress, as well as a pull to be nurtured and taken care of by the examiner. Meersand (2011) outlines diverse transferential responses that children exhibit, including seeing the testing as punishment for being bad, believing in the magical powers of the tester to perceive their faults, and fear that the test will reveal hidden thoughts or damage. The child may also have benign views of the tester, who can be perceived as a helpful and supportive adult. Sandler (1995) describes the testing situation as a potentially "safe space" where children can feel encouraged; their self-esteem may improve upon receiving positive reinforcement and attention. For example, the tester can complement children on a job well done, engage with them in a game, and attend to their feelings in the situation.

THE TESTER'S RESPONSE TO THE PARENT AND CHILD

The tester also brings countertransferential feelings to the testing experience, which may distort his or her understanding of the child or how best to communicate testing results. Countertransferential reactions to children can include anxiety surrounding the introduction of difficult tasks, impatience, and frustration when the child is impulsive or oppositional, and a strong desire to help and protect the child. Sugarman (1981) delineates diverse manifestations of countertransference in the testing situation and advocates using these responses as another lens through which to understand the child. Frustration on the part of the tester can be indicative of the child's difficulty with aggression. Similarly, feelings of anxiety on the part of the tester can signal concordant anxiety of the child. Chused (1988) noted that children's helplessness may arouse guilt or regret in the clinician for presenting challenging tasks that lead the child to struggle. When children are impulsive and/or oppositional, the tester may feel fatigued and frustrated.

Just as the tester experiences countertransference feelings towards the child, he or she can also experience countertransference to the parents. The tester may feel intimidated by the parents and may perceive information about the child as potentially threatening to them. The tester may feel warmly towards the family and want to shield them from "bad news," or might soft-pedal the results in a way that downplays the severity of the child's problems. Countertransferential reactions on the tester's part can also include anxiety with regard to how the parents view the tester, frustration with the parents when they do not agree with the results, envy of the parents for their perceived status (financial and otherwise) and feeling intimidated by parents' intense emotions. The therapist should be aware of these themes as they may impact the family's experience of the testing.

SELF-DISCLOSURE

I will now discuss the use of self-disclosure when working with patients with neurocognitive challenges. Self-disclosure is an example of therapists using their own experiences to help the patient. Self-disclosure is an aspect of the transference/countertransference matrix, as it is directly related to the therapists' internal experience and can arouse strong transferential feelings in the patient and/or family. The therapist must be mindful of the impact on the transference when he or she chooses to self-disclose. I posit that therapists' self-disclosure of their own neurocognitive disorders is a powerful way to help the patient come to terms with their neurocognitive challenges. I will now present a brief literature review of self-disclosure along with case examples of using this technique to intervene effectively with neurocognitive challenges.

LITERATURE REVIEW

Self-disclosure is a modern issue; in the early years of psychoanalysis, Freud (1912) famously declared that the therapist should be a blank screen. He advocated nondisclosure on the therapist's part and even indicated that the patient's frustration with the therapist's opaqueness was essential to the treatment. Freud saw the therapeutic relationship as a psychological model in which the focus rests solely on the patient; the curative aspect of the treatment would therefore emerge from the patient's own insights into his or her symptoms. Despite this proclamation, the reality of the analytic situation did not live up to the expressed ideal. Freud's patients were privy to information about him and his family. He was known to give gifts to his patients and to take walks with them. Certainly, his decision to analyze his own daughter, Anna Freud, contradicts his idea of the blank screen. Despite these discrepancies, Freudian analysis promotes the notion that in order to better encourage fantasies and the uncovering of unconscious material, the analyst must never volunteer personal information.

As psychoanalysis evolved, many theorists turned their attention to the patient-therapist relationship as a key factor in the treatment. Mitchell (1988), the foremost proponent of relational theory, proposed a "two-person model" of analysis, such that the therapist and patient have mutual influence on each other, and intervention is understood within that matrix. This model conceptualizes therapist self-disclosure as an aspect of the analytic work. This idea dates back to Ferenczi's (1928) proposal of mutual analysis for therapist and patient. Although Ferenczi's bold prescription was not adopted by psychoanalysts, the perils and possibilities of self-disclosure began to be addressed both in the clinical setting and in the analytic literature.

In Aron's view (1991), self-disclosure is simply unavoidable: "[S]elf revelation is not an option for the analyst, it is an inevitability." (Aron, 1991, p.40). He expounds on how deliberate self-disclosure can take many forms: disclosure of feelings, personal information, and so on. Perhaps the most obvious disadvantage of deliberate self-disclosure is its potential to obscure the patient's experiences in favor of the therapist's as will be discussed in more detail below. On the other hand, therapist self-disclosure can confirm patients' sense of reality and establish the therapist as empathic. Basescu (1990) proposes that engaging the patient as a collaborator by giving them access to the analyst's experience facilitates the treatment. Likewise, Ehrenberg (1992) believes all treatments can be advanced by deliberate self-disclosure of affect.

Similarly, Aron (1996) noted that patients desire to know their therapist the way children long to understand their parents; thus, the analytic work should include information about the therapist for the patient. At the same time, therapists must ensure that their needs remain independent of the patient's, much like a parent who needs to carve out his or her personal time away from their children. Hence, withholding information is sometimes, if not always, the correct course of action.

Menaker (1990) commented that when the "analyst reveals something about him or herself, it becomes an echo of the patient's own experience and thus serves to cement the bond between patient and therapist." Authenticity in the analyst facilitates the patient's development of his or herself. Menaker cautions that therapeutic self-disclosure must always be motivated by regard for the patient's development. If the self-disclosure misfires, those situations provide an opportunity to explore with the patient what went wrong and improve communication.

Some types of self-disclosure are inevitable and unavoidable: therapists' skin color and name, whether they wear a wedding band, their internet presence, their choice of office and manner of attire—even the presence of pregnancy. Other information can be more easily hidden, such as sexual orientation, ethnicity, learning and attention deficits, psychiatric disorders, and medical illnesses. Disclosing hidden aspects of identity renders the therapist vulnerable and can be seen as controversial. In a sense, it is similar to coming out to patients as gay, lesbian, or trans—as these types of identities are often hidden and/or stigmatized (Satterly, 2006; Thomas, 2008). At the same time, the therapist can be a powerful role model for the patient who is struggling with similar issues, both in terms of coping with the challenges of these identities and in terms of not buying into the culture of shame and secrecy.

SELF-DISCLOSURE OF A LEARNING DISABILITY

I maintain that when the therapist self discloses about a shameful aspect of his or her identity, in this case, having a learning disability, this can ease the pain and shame for the patient who has a similar presentation. Establishing oneself as a role model and a person with whom to identify regarding a similar area of challenge can help patients feel less alone and less humiliated by their perceived inadequacies. Of course, a therapist can establish him or herself as a role model that resonates with the patient and helps the patient tolerate and work through feelings of shame without having had a similar experience or self-disclosing about the experience. Nonetheless, I suggest that directly presenting yourself as an object with whom to identify is especially helpful in those situations where shame is a predominant emotion.

As noted above, shame is a common and understandable reaction to the stigma surrounding learning disabilities and the many experiences of failure associated with them. As Aron (2013) points out, "Because it is so often concealed from view, shame is considered a hidden emotion." As shame has a tendency to go underground, it is essential that the therapist remain attuned to these feelings, both in the patient and the therapist. Responding to my patients' recounting of shameful experiences by merely listening might actually make them more embarrassed by insinuating that their painful experiences are not being tolerated by the therapist. I would take this perspective even further and posit that the therapist's self-disclosure reduces shame in the patient.

I have a nonverbal learning disability that significantly interfered with my math skills in elementary school. There was a large discrepancy between my low math skills and highly developed reading skills that persisted throughout high school. As I was undiagnosed and unremediated, I only realized my learning issues when I applied to graduate school. I often share my experiences in elementary school, particularly with parents, to help them understand the experiences of a bright child with uneven performance caused by learning disorders. This offers the family hope and can help destigmatize the diagnosis. When I do so, I have noticed that parents will then often share their similar experiences with me, leading to increased empathy for their child. With patients, I will also share my experiences both as a role model to help them understand that they can succeed and compensate for their learning issues as well as a way to mitigate some of the shame and distress that comes along with the disorder. The following case examples illustrate the benefits and pitfalls of self-disclosure of a learning disability.

A bright, verbal 11-year-old girl was diagnosed with dyscalculia. She teared up as she recounted her struggles with math, and feelings of frustration and concerns that she was "stupid." I empathized with her feelings and shared my own challenges with math. I told her that we could come up with strategies that would help her better understand the material; I assured her that she would be able to succeed despite her disability. As we talked, she brightened, and she left the session feeling more confident about her academic future.

Another example illustrates the nuances of self-disclosure in long-term treatment. A patient with a significant history of LD was discussing her anxiety about applying to graduate programs. When I commiserated, she said sharply

> and accusatorily, "What do you know about applications to graduate school? You had to apply three times before you got accepted." I was taken aback by her accusation; I had shared my experiences of rejection by graduate schools with my patients as a cautionary tale to reflect on how persistence will help you achieve your goals. Now she was shaming me for my experience and telling me I was inadequate and could not help her. I took a deep breath and reflected, "Oh that's very interesting that you see it that way, I have never looked at it that way but I can see what you are saying." This admission and tolerance of my own shame softened her stance and she began discussing her fears that she would not get into school and that she would not be able to perform when she got there. In this instance, accepting and metabolizing the shame helped her move beyond her shame and discuss her fears.

Self-disclosure needs to be seen as something offered that is therapeutic and patient centered. Among the pitfalls of using this technique is that the patient may feel put off, that you are sharing too much information and that you are hijacking the session to talk about yourself. Likewise, the patient may feel intruded upon by you sharing your vulnerabilities. They may feel that you are "over sharing" and lose confidence in the therapeutic process. They may also have less confidence in you if they know you have a learning disability, and they may devalue you the way they devalue themselves. In addition, the patient may feel alienated and misunderstood if you are advocating a different response than the one, they have taken. Self-disclosure needs to be executed in a sensitive and cautious manner with the awareness that you may be falling into one of the above traps. A clinical exchange further illustrates both the challenges and possibilities of self-disclosure of learning disabilities.

> A long-standing patient was frustrated by my perceived lack of understanding about her situation and called me a "dumb-ass bitch." I pointed out to her that I did not think I was "dumb" in any way. She retorted "But you have a learning disability, that makes you stupid." This led to an extremely productive conversation regarding her feelings about her own learning difficulties, past experiences in a mainstream school that painfully contributed to herself perception as stupid, and an awareness that you can be intelligent and still have learning disabilities.

Self-disclosure can also be useful when discussing recommendations for services as well as strategies that the patient and the family can use to improve skills and functioning. If I have had personal experience with any of the service providers or use any of the strategies, I will often offer my experiences to help the patient understand the efficacy of the interventions.

Similarly, I may also tell them about other patients' experiences with the modalities, providers, or strategies to help them understand their benefits. Reassuring patients and their families that they are not alone in the struggle and that there is effective intervention available facilitates trust, acceptance of the recommendations and positive outcomes.

The following case example illustrates the potentially reassuring effect of this type of self-disclosure.

> In a parent guidance session, my patient discussed a dilemma with parenting her daughter who has ADD and often lies to take the "easy way out." I commiserated with her situation and shared that my teenage son with ADD also exhibits similar behaviors. I did not want her to feel I was preaching or unsympathetic as I urged her to be understanding of her daughter's issues and refrain from being overly punitive and rigid. Sharing my struggle enabled her to relax, chuckle and display more insight and self-reflection. Using myself as a model and a flawed one at that opened up the conversation for one of sharing and commiseration.

To recap, disclosing this type of personal information puts the therapist in a vulnerable position and can be seen as controversial. In a sense, it is similar to coming out to patients as gay, lesbian, or transgender—as these types of identities are often seen as hidden or stigmatized (Satterly, 2006; Thomas, 2008) At the same time, the therapist can be a powerful role model for the patient who is struggling with similar issues both in terms of coping with the challenges of these identities and in terms of not buying into the culture of shame and secrecy surrounding these issues.

In conclusion, working with patients with neurocognitive challenges can elicit intense transferential/countertransferential responses. Patients may view the therapist as a judgmental, critical authority figure who is disappointed by their poor performance. Therapists may feel bewildered and frustrated by the impact of the neurocognitive deficits on the treatment and the patient's defensiveness regarding intervention. Therapeutic strategies include understanding the neurocognitive etiology of these disruptions to treatment, demonstrating compassion, and understanding to the patients and understanding that integrating the learning disorder and past history of painfully shaming experiences into a positive sense of self is a long and painstaking process. In addition, for those therapists who also struggle with neurocognitive challenges and who have succeeded professionally despite such difficulties, self-disclosure can be an effective strategy to dispel shame and facilitate self-acceptance in their patients.

Chapter Eight

The Impact of COVID-19 and Remote Learning on Patients with ADD, LD, and Autism

The COVID-19 pandemic led to many months of school closures, quarantine, and social isolation for children and their families. This disruption of routine has had significant implications for the mental health of children and adolescents, leading to a parallel mental health pandemic among this vulnerable population (Fegert, 2020). While these psychosocial effects were most acute during the initial phase, the ripples of the pandemic continue to be felt even years after its onset, as we continue to be confronted with the ever-evolving virus and its myriad aftereffects. A review of the literature suggests an increase in depression and anxiety among children and adolescents during the pandemic as a result of the sweeping changes to their environment (Waite et al., 2020; Vizard et al., 2020; Berendese, 2021). Fear of contagion, boredom, loneliness, increased social anxiety, irritability, inattention, and increased disruptive behaviors were all observed (de Figueiredo, 2021; Jiao et al., 2020). For children with neurocognitive impairments, the impact was even more severe (Korpa, 2021) due to a proliferation of factors that will be discussed below. Nonetheless, despite the pandemic's pointed impact on mental health, some children and adolescents were actually able to thrive and even experienced improvements in their social and emotional functioning (Chawla et al., 2021; Silk et al., 2022).

For adults with autism, the impact of COVID contributed to varying degrees of deterioration in mental health. A survey of autistic people in the UK indicated that disruption of normal routines and uncertainty about the future caused anxiety and depression (Davidson et al., 2021). A mixed method approach using data from three countries confirmed these findings. Adults with autism showed a greater increase in worries about their pets, work, getting medication and food, and their own safety/security. While they felt relieved from ordinary social stresses, they still experienced the loss of social contact as difficult (Oomen et al., 2021).

For adults with ADHD, symptom severity appeared to be exacerbated during the COVID-19 pandemic. Self-ratings confirmed increased depression and social isolation (Sibley et al., 2021). Similarly, a survey of 238 males with ADD pointed to an increase in anxiety, depression, inattentiveness, and hyperactive/impulsive behaviors (Breaux et al., 2021).

Regarding college students with learning disabilities, survey data indicated a significant decline in mental and physical health and educational expectations during the pandemic (Halpern-Manners et al., 2022). In contrast, interviews of 609 adults with learning disabilities explored both worries/negative outcomes and positive outcomes from the COVID-19 pandemic. Social isolation was the most commonly reported worry/negative along with changes to/loss of routine, loss of support/services and decreased health/well-being/fitness. Some positive aspects included access to community on the computer, more time spent with family, improved health/well-being/fitness, and a slower pace of life. (Flynn et al., 2021). Thus, COVID contributed to significant mental health issues but also provided some benefits among adults with neurocognitive disorders.

The pandemic also had considerable impact on children's academic functioning, resulting in a deterioration in functioning termed the COVID "slide," that is, a regression in academic performance due to remote learning (Hoofman & Secord, 2021). In 2022, for the first time since the National Assessment of Educational Progress tests began tracking student achievement in the 1970s, 9-year-olds lost ground in math (Mervosh, 2023). In addition, reading scores fell by the largest margin in more than 30 years. The declines spanned almost all races and income levels and were markedly worse for the lowest-performing students. While top performers (in the 90th percentile or above) showed a modest drop of only 3 points, students in the bottom 10th percentile dropped 12 points, indicating four times the impact (Mervosh, 2022).

There are many factors contributing both to the decline in mental health and academic success. First, the loss of physical activity and increase in sedentary behaviors (particularly involving screen time) contributed to depression, poor academic achievement, impaired cardiovascular health, and obesity (Xiang et al., 2020). Second, the loss of the school routine has been linked to increased anxiety and depression (Lee, 202). Third, social isolation hits children and adolescents harder, as their development is inextricably connected to socialization and peer relationships. Adolescence is a time of deep learning about the social environment and "virtual contact" disrupts this learning (de Figueiredo, 2021; Torres et al., 2021). Additionally, reduced access to support services including medication, therapy, and specialized instruction devastated children and teens in need of such services (Serlachius, 2020).

LEARNING DISORDERS

The so-called "COVID slide" is significantly greater for those children at social or educational risk, as they may regress especially intensely without in-person instruction (Sharfstein, 2020), leading to anxiety, depression, frustration, and lowered self-esteem (Korpa, 2021). The relationship between lowered academic achievement and depression and anxiety is well-documented (Peluso, 2005). A negative cycle develops, with academic struggles leading to learned helplessness, which leads to avoidance, which leads to further academic difficulties that ultimately contribute to mental health problems (Masten et al., 2005; Valås, 2021).

Children with language-based learning disorders require specialized instruction to help them attain academic proficiency, particularly with reading and writing. They often require special education classes with access to diverse teaching methods, such as the Orton-Gillingham approach for reading (Ritchey et al., 2006). Delivery of these services relies on a direct instruction approach; this entails a method of explicit teaching involving goal setting, frequent rehearsal of the material, chunking the material into small bits, and scaffolding the curriculum in orderly sequences with frequent evaluation of skills (Adams & Engleman, 1996). The individualized nature of this teaching method is extremely difficult to replicate on Zoom. Thus, many children who were receiving special education services were not able to obtain adequate instruction during the pandemic and consequently fell behind.

In addition, children with language-based learning disorders often demonstrate social challenges, as they have difficulty comprehending complicated social interactions or keeping up with the rapid banter of peers (Bryan, 1991). Social isolation exacerbates these deficits, leading to increased loneliness and social anxiety. A case example illustrates this phenomenon.

> Sarah, a 12-year-old girl, was referred for therapy by her parents who cited concerns about moodiness and irritability. She had been diagnosed with dyslexia and attended a special education school. She described feeling increasingly left out socially during the pandemic and said she could not keep up with her peers on social media. She poignantly described significant anxiety with regard to reaching out to peers, as she lacked the structure of the classroom and the classroom routines that used to facilitate such interactions.

Children with nonverbal learning disorders are also significantly impacted by the social isolation imposed during the pandemic, as the lack of access to peers and cues exacerbates their vulnerability to psychosocial difficulties. Their right hemisphere impairments compromise their understanding of the social gestalt, and they require practice and experience to progress in their mastery of social pragmatics and nuance. Thus, lack of exposure atrophies their already compromised social skills and stunts any further progress in the social sphere.

ATTENTION DISORDERS

The deficits in executive functioning associated with ADD render the organization of tasks and time management excruciatingly difficult for children and teens with attentional disorders (Barkley, 2018). Thus, the pandemic-related disruption of routine and loss of structure only added to these challenges. In addition, as schooling was provided primarily via Zoom, children with ADD found it even more difficult to focus on school. The home environment is more distracting than school and video education is less compelling than personal interaction. Further, lack of physical activity is a significant contributor to lowered mood, as exercise has been proven to improve depression and anxiety (Peluso, 2005).

Children with ADHD who are motorically restless suffer particularly from a lack of scheduled sports and outdoor time. These children rely on athletic outlets to channel their energy in a constructive manner, which enhances their attention to schoolwork while in the classroom. In a survey of children with ADHD during the pandemic, researchers found both decreased exercise and outdoor time and increased anxiety, depression, television use, and loneliness compared with the period before the lockdown. In general, these children reported more stress and poorer overall functioning (Sciberras et al., 2020). A case example illustrates the challenges of children with ADD during the pandemic:

Carter, an 8-year-old boy, was referred for an assessment by his parents at the request of his school. The presenting problems included poor academic achievement, oppositionality, and withdrawal from activities. Carter's parents recounted that, prior to the pandemic, he was a lively and energetic boy who was impulsive but also cheerful and cooperative. However, he could not seem to attend to Zoom learning and could only focus if an adult was sitting next to him—which was not always possible. Carter expressed frustration with his academic tasks and said that school was "hard" and "boring." He missed his friends and going to class. Carter was diagnosed with ADD and began medication and teletherapy, which facilitated a better adjustment to school.

Children with attention disorders often demonstrate social deficits due to their impulsivity, difficulty attending to cues, and general distractibility (Osman, 1995). Social isolation further exacerbates these issues, as children miss out on the experience and modeling required to improve upon their social skills. Taken together, social isolation, lowered academic performance, and a lack of physical activity all contribute to increased levels of anxiety, depression, loneliness, and low self-esteem.

Lastly, children with ADD are more vulnerable to acquiring an addiction to computers due to their sensitivity to immediate feedback and instant gratification, poor frustration tolerance, and need for activity (Biolauc et al., 2008). Reliance on the computer for academic and social interaction intensifies these addictive tendencies as, in the context of remote learning, there is always a reason to be on the computer. Indeed, in my own practice, I have noted a significant increase of parents referring their children for screen addiction or describing challenges in removing their children from electronics during the pandemic.

AUTISM SPECTRUM DISORDER

Loss of a regular routine is extremely challenging for children with autism spectrum disorder, as they have a particular aversion to change and transition. In addition, they are heavily reliant on supportive services to facilitate functioning due to their impaired interpersonal skills, difficulty with change/disruption of routine, and poor tolerance of sensory and emotional stimulation. They are thus easily destabilized by changes in their services. Further, staying at home with their families—who may either not fully understand their special needs or be poorly equipped to cope with them—adds another significant challenge to these children's well-being. In fact, a survey of families who care for children with ASD revealed that the most significant stressor for their children was disruption of the daily routine (White et al., 2021). In addition, due to their tendency toward obsessional thinking, children and adolescents with autism often harbor significant health-related anxieties. Likewise, COVID-related fears (many exaggerated and unrealistic) were prominent among this population (Kalvin et al., 2021).

A case example illustrates the impact of COVID-19 and lockdown on a high functioning teen with autism:

> Adam, a bright, articulate 16-year-old boy with autism spectrum disorder, was referred for treatment due to his withdrawal from academic and social activities. His parents reported that, prior to COVID-19, he attended a mainstream school and had a limited circle of friends with whom he had regular social contact. When school went remote, Adam withdrew. Previously an accomplished student, he nearly failed all his classes. He also refused to socialize

with peers or family members. He even became distressed when his parents hired a repairman and responded by staying in his room for the majority of the day. In treatment, he spoke poignantly of his fears of getting sick or infecting others. He was convinced he had a suppressed immune system, although there was no medical evidence to support this belief. In addition, he expressed the idea that people with disabilities (such as himself and his friends) were more at risk during COVID-19, though again there was no medical support for this assertion.

SILVER LINING

Despite the significant and pervasive difficulties presented by COVID for children and adolescents with neurocognitive disorders, some beneficial effects have been noted. Firstly, increased family time was linked to improved well-being among children and families (Sciberras et al., 2022). Parents also reported improved eating and sleeping among children during lockdown, possibly as a result of increased parental supervision (Łuszczki et al., 2021). For many families, life dramatically slowed down and there was an almost total reliance on the family unit as the primary source of social interaction and support. These factors had the potential to strengthen family bonds and reduce stress for children and their parents. Decreased pressure from school and other activities and increased time with family and for pursuits such as leisure reading, hobbies, and music were also noted as positive effects (Silk. et al., 2022). Further, not meeting in person in school reduces the risk of bullying, which is a significant stressor for children with special needs (Zablotsky et al., 2013). We might speculate that children who were more introverted or socially anxious were able to appreciate the reduced social pressure, whereas more extroverted children missed their peers and social interaction at school. A case example will illustrate this idea:

Sarah, a poised and verbal 13-year-old girl with dyslexia and ADD, had a habit of yelling loudly whenever she was distressed or agitated. Her outbursts were extremely difficult to contain and alienated her from family members. During the pandemic, she spent several uninterrupted months with her mother in the countryside. This experience was very therapeutic for Sarah as she had her mother's undivided attention as well as additional support for her classwork. Eventually, her mother noticed that Sarah had completely stopped her outbursts during this period, which she credited to a decrease in Sarah's anxiety. Sarah also reported improved mastery of her academic skills.

INTERVENTIONS

I will now discuss therapeutic strategies for children, adolescents, and adults with each type of disorder to maximize their adaptation to the myriad challenges presented by the COVID-19 pandemic.

Individuals with nonverbal learning disorders are verbal and articulate but have difficulty performing visual-spatial tasks, such as reading diagrams or maps. Organization and time management challenges are also part of this disorder. As students transition to online learning, their ability to stay organized and engaged with their schoolwork could be particularly challenged due to the loss of routine and support in school. The therapist could offer help by creating an online calendar, encouraging patients to share their goals with parents, teachers, or tutors by emailing them about goals and meeting with them individually to review their work. The therapist can also recommend organizational strategies for effective learning and coordination of materials, such as using graphic organizers, bullet journaling (instead of blank, lined pages, the bullet journal contains specific sections to log daily to-dos, keep a calendar, jot down notes, track physical and mental health, and record goals), and using alarms to keep themselves on track.

Individuals with language-based learning disorders have difficulty expressing themselves; they often become tongue tied in social and academic situations. As mentioned above, losing the access to social cues and experience can further atrophy their social skills. The therapist could help by role-playing situations, finding online forums for socialization, and encouraging patients to advocate for their needs with peers and teachers. Online art therapy groups using WhatsApp have also proven an effective intervention to combat social isolation during the pandemic (Datlen & Pandolfi, 2020).

Children and adolescents with ADD also suffer from social and academic challenges. Their high level of distractibility and lack of focus makes it painful to initiate and complete academic tasks. In addition, they can inadvertently offend peers with their tangential conversation and disinhibited comments. Online learning exacerbates these challenges and heightens the propensity to be self-critical and frustrated with poor achievement. The therapist could help by brainstorming strategies for effective learning and finding online forums for support. Highlighting their areas of strength and emphasizing their abilities to adapt to their challenges is also important and facilitates self-confidence and productivity.

Adults with ADD also reported increased symptoms during COVID, including social isolation, boredom, and motivation problems. Recommended interventions include reducing risk factors by increasing social interaction and helping adults with ADD engage in productive behaviors, such as exercise, engaging in hobbies, and forming relationships (Sibley et al., 2021). A study comparing telepsychiatry with on-site sessions using face masks with adult ADD patients indicated no difference in the quality of the sessions or therapeutic alliance. Patients and therapists identified positive effects as well as challenges with both modalities (Wyler et al., 2021).

As noted above, for individuals with autism spectrum disorder, the specific challenges of COVID-19 can be devastating—particularly the disruption of routines and lack of access to services. The therapist can help by encouraging adherence to routines, facilitating compliance with online platforms, and helping them take advantage of online resources. Individuals with autistic spectrum disorder have the potential to excel when presented with online platforms as they often respond positively to the structure of these platforms.

The following case example illustrates use of these techniques.

Alex, a young adult with ASD and anxiety, manifested significant symptoms related to COVID-19. He became severely phobic about leaving the house and worried he would infect others. He continued to do his schooling online but demonstrated obsessive worrying about COVID-19; he reduced his socializing dramatically and even preferred to eat meals away from his parents, citing concerns about their health. In treatment, I discussed the etiology of his concerns, emphasizing how his ASD interferes with his ability to organize his day, comply with academic tasks, and keep up socially—even online. We outlined a daily schedule and implemented "bullet journaling" to assist with goal implementation. The bullet journal method is a checklist of key goals to accomplish during the day that facilitates motivation and accountability. The journal also includes sections to log daily tasks, keep a monthly or weekly calendar, jot down notes and record both short term and long-term goals. The use of organizational techniques and better recognition of the impact of his neurocognitive impairments reduced Alex's anxiety and improved his ability to complete tasks. He was able to complete his courses, begin to go outside again, and socialize with peers online.

MODIFICATION OF HEALTHCARE INTERVENTIONS: TURNING TO TELEMEDICINE

The provision of mental health services changed dramatically during the pandemic. Telemedicine proliferated as lockdown greatly impacted access to the types of healthcare resources, such as therapy, medication, and other clinical services that children with special needs require (Brandenburg et al., 2020). Psychiatrists, psychologists, and occupational and speech therapists all turned to telemedicine as the primary modality of service delivery. With creativity and ingenuity, services were delivered to those young people in need, and the majority of patients ascribe benefit to such services (Brandenburg et al., 2020). However, the quality of telemedicine can be variable in vulnerable populations, such as economically disadvantaged children, who face even more barriers to care during COVID-19.

As demonstrated above, there was an increased need for mental health services during the COVID-19 pandemic. Concomitantly, delivery of services was disrupted by the lockdown as the transition to the home as a primary base for school and work became the norm for most people. Telemedicine became the dominant vehicle for delivering mental health services. A review of the literature demonstrates the effectiveness of teletherapy for children with special needs, along with its specific challenges (McCullough, 2001; Tse, 2015). Clinical as well as research-based data indicate that teletherapy can ameliorate symptoms and improve mental health. Telemedicine can be challenging to deliver, however, as there may be lack of space or privacy at home (Sharma & Bhaskar, 2020). Additionally, play therapy (particularly with young children) can be a daunting task to accomplish over Zoom. Enlisting parents to facilitate the therapy was one solution to this problem.

Maier et al. (2021) and Narvaez et al. (2022) note the benefits of telemedicine and outline specific strategies to render teletherapy effective. These benefits include greater flexibility in scheduling, which allows for more consistent and regular sessions; greater ability to include multiple family members and caregivers in the sessions; and the opportunity for parent management training. Specific strategies for maximizing effectiveness include offering incentives for participation, such as encouraging the child to share a favorite video or pet online; offering technology rewards, such as virtual stickers; use of the "teach" features of video conferencing, such as shared screen, video chat, or drawing or writing with the patient; and setting a screen agenda with online timers. Two case examples illustrate the benefits of online therapy during the pandemic:

> Nancy, an exuberant 5-year-old girl, was referred for therapy due to significant anxiety and distress, particularly regarding her parents' separation. Her symptoms coalesced around difficulty with sleeping and continuous fighting with her siblings. Treatment was conducted online as a result of the pandemic. I was able to easily engage Nancy with the squiggle game using the shared screen to draw and create stories together. Nancy then requested art supplies from her parents and began to create pictures and tell me stories that revealed her fears of loss and abandonment. We worked together on these themes and saved the pictures and stories, either digitally or on paper. On the computer, she held up her pictures, I then took pictures of her art and typed the stories on the computer. Stories and drawings were also stored on paper in her bedroom.

At the end of several months, Nancy's symptoms alleviated, and she presented with improved sleep and reduced conflict with siblings.

Aaron, a 16-year-old boy with high-functioning autism, was referred for online therapy during the pandemic due to significant anxiety and depression. Individual remote therapy worked well for Aaron, as he discussed his fears related to COVID-19, anxiety related to social isolation, and difficulty maintaining a consistent routine. Teletherapy also allowed Aaron to share his hobbies with me, for example showing me a sweater he was knitting, or even introducing me to his cat on Zoom. This ability to visually share his life helped Aaron connect effectively with me, which was especially valuable as he has significant social communication difficulties due to his autism. When Aaron became distressed, however, he asked me to text with him, as he was finding it difficult to speak and felt too overwhelmed and emotional to talk; his low tolerance of affective stimulation and the fragility of his communication abilities are central challenges of his autism. Fortunately, we successfully resolved his concerns via text. The use of texting instead of talking is specific to remote therapy and, in this case, created a valuable forum for Aaron to air his concerns.

Regarding the impact on therapists, telemedicine was a lifesaver in that it allowed therapeutic work to continue albeit under very different circumstances. In addition, many therapists appreciate the convenience and flexibility that remote sessions offer. However, telemedicine has also been associated with "screen fatigue" as well as difficulty maintaining focus and engaging on an intense affective level. Seemingly all agree that it takes a significant physical and emotional toll to conduct therapy via video or telephone (Markowitz, 2021; Reese et al., 2002). A survey of high school students and training therapists found equivalent challenges despite widespread agreement that the therapy was overall effective (Sehon, 2015). Personally, I find it difficult to maintain engagement during online sessions, and it takes more energy to maintain focus as compared with in-person sessions. Challenges also include an overly casual approach by patients during sessions, as many patients may talk with their therapists in their beds or even lying down. In addition, people and pets may come into the sessions, and both patients and therapists may be distracted by emails, texts, and online entertainment that are visible or easily accessible on the computer screen (Markowitz, 2021).

RIPPLE EFFECT

Although the most severe phases of COVID-19 have passed (i.e., we are out of lockdown, we have vaccines and masking is optional in many spaces), we continue to grapple with its impact—particularly regarding academic progress and the mental health of children, adolescents, and adults. For individuals with neurocognitive challenges, the impact has been much more significant, given their vulnerabilities as discussed above. For most individuals with neurocognitive disorders, COVID-19 worsened their symptoms due to the social isolation and anxiety related to the epidemic. Therefore, clinicians need to be attentive to this population's needs and design specific interventions to ameliorate COVID's ongoing impact.

Chapter Nine

Race, Culture, and Socioeconomic Status

Factors in Diagnosis and Intervention with Patients with Neurocognitive Challenges

Race, culture, and socioeconomic status play a role in assessment and intervention with patients with neurocognitive challenges. In this chapter, I will discuss the implications of these factors regarding specific learning and attention disorders. I will also offer suggestions for best practices, including becoming culturally informed and taking into account one's own biases when working with multicultural families. I will begin with discussing cultural concerns when performing neuropsychological assessments and then delve into each disorder and implications for treatment.

CULTURAL CONCERNS IN NEUROPSYCHOLOGICAL ASSESSMENTS

When diagnosing and creating a unique learning profile, it is critical to keep in mind the cultural and bilingual concerns that can impact the testing and recommendations. If a child or adult is bilingual, it is important to assess in both languages in order to properly gauge his or her functioning. It is also imperative to understand different cultures regarding expectations for behavior and responses to tests. Additionally, certain test items are culturally biased and need to be interpreted in that light. For example, the Thematic Apperception Test, a projective test of personality, only features images of white people drawn in the 1930s. Further, tests that assess social judgment, fund of information, and vocabulary are particularly skewed toward majority cultural and linguistic assumptions. For example, the historical facts reference European or North American items, and the social judgment questions reflect the norms and values of the majority culture.

Race and class differences can engender anxiety among parents and children and render the testing, especially stressful for minority and low-income families because the professionals who are working with them may come from dissimilar cultural, racial and class backgrounds. Therefore, they may feel misunderstood and uncomfortable as their culture is not reflected in the testing. When a child is uncomfortable, the test results may be compromised and reflect lower performance than is necessarily the case. As a psychologist working for the Board of Education in a poor, non-white neighborhood, I witnessed countless examples of disrespect and intimidation by the teachers and administration towards the children and their families. These encounters led the children to mistrust white authority figures and underperform when being evaluated.

Sensitivity to socioeconomic considerations includes tailoring the recommendations to accommodate financial concerns. The tester needs to be mindful of the family's resources and provide information that is appropriate for the family. In-network recommendations should be made when the family can only afford those options. Recommendations for educational lawyers and advocates to assist families are particularly useful for families that could not otherwise afford special education services for their children. They recover the legal fees from the city as well as the tuition.

Mindt et al. (2008) recommend best practices for providing neuropsychological services for patients of a different race/ethnicity from the clinician or from the majority culture, including using the most culturally sensitive instruments available—that is, relying on nonverbal tests to measure intelligence, and acknowledging the limitations of the tests and norms in the findings. In addition, the examiner should gather as much sociocultural information as possible to best contextualize the results. Best practices also include referring to a neuropsychologist with expertise with these clients when possible and to be actively involved in professional activities to advance cultural competence.

I will now discuss each disorder regarding prevalence of the disorder, etiology of racial and cultural discrepancies and specific intervention techniques designed for cultural sensitivity.

ATTENTION DEFICIT HYPERACTIVITY DISORDER (ADHD)

Prevalence

When I began my practice in the 1990s, parents often reacted with shock and horror to a diagnosis of ADHD for their child. These days (i.e., 2023), I often have children as young as 11 or 12 come into my office and confidently announce that they have ADHD. They are usually correct, and their parents typically accept the diagnosis in a well-adjusted manner and add statements such as, "I always knew it." This clinical observation mirrors the statistics on ADHD. The estimated number of children aged three to 17 years diagnosed with ADHD is about six million (9.8%), according to a national survey of parents (Bitsko et al., 2022). In a national survey of physician office visits and medication prescriptions, diagnoses of ADHD increased by 36 percent in adults and 18 percent in youths from 2008–2013. However, ADHD diagnosis was 77 percent less likely among black children as compared to white youths in 2012–2013 (Fairman et al., 2020).

Several large epidemiological studies found white children to receive ADHD diagnoses and treatment more than black, Hispanic and Asian children (Danielson et al., 2018; Shi, 2021; Wong & Landes, 2022). In the Shi study, all children were covered by commercial insurance, so we can assume they had equal access to health care. What are some of the variables responsible for this phenomenon of underdiagnosis and treatment of ADHD among minority children? Several factors, including income differentials, varying cultural norms, and practitioner bias, have been implicated in this problem.

ETIOLOGY OF ETHNIC/RACIAL DISPARITIES

Socioeconomic Status/Access to Healthcare

Socioeconomic status has been identified as a major obstacle to proper diagnosis and treatment of ADHD, as evaluation and treatment is expensive and often requires multiple visits to diverse practitioners, including psychiatrists and psychologists. Thus, lower income families with less access to health care are at a disadvantage in getting effective intervention. Likewise, children without insurance had lower levels of care in data from the 1997–2000 Medical Expenditure Panel Survey (Stevens et al., 2005). Nonwhite and immigrant groups are more likely than white families to fall into low-income groups, such that ethnicity and socioeconomic status are powerfully entwined.

Parental Perceptions/Cultural Norms

It has been suggested that parents' perceptions of disorders or available services may play a role in the underdiagnosis and treatment of minority children. In a multi-site sample of 4,297 children, many black parents rated their children to demonstrate ADHD symptoms on parent questionnaires, although these children had received neither clinical diagnosis nor treatment (Coker et al., 2016). What factors might influence parental reluctance to diagnose their children with ADHD? Firstly, parents might distrust the system, and their concerns about racism may affect their willingness to approach the health care system (Trent et al., 2019). Secondly, minority parents may distrust medication and feel reluctant to use medication to "control" their children (Carpenter-Song, 2008).

Several studies specifically address black parents' attitudes towards medication. One study highlighting this concern among African American families surveyed parents of children treated for ADHD in an urban primary care setting. Over two thirds (71%) of these families were initially hesitant to use stimulants (dosReis et al., 2006). Similarly, Schnittker (2003) found that compared to white families, African American families were more concerned about the use of psychotropic medications to treat their children, less likely to believe they are effective, more likely to be concerned with side effects, and less likely to give medication to their children.

In addition, fear of social stigma was found to be more prevalent among ethnic minority families (Slobodin & Masalha, 2020). Persistent concern exists about the over-pathologizing of African American and other minority children, especially boys. Minority families were more likely to ascribe attention problems to personality variables as compared with seeking a diagnosis based on symptoms (Alvarado & Modesto-Lowe, 2017).

Practitioner Bias

Practitioner bias has also been implicated in the underdiagnosis and reduced intervention for ADHD among minority youth. A review of studies assessing "real world" diagnostic practice suggest that black children may be over diagnosed with Oppositional Defiant Disorder (ODD), despite epidemiological literature indicating similar prevalence of ODD and ADHD across racial groups (Ballentine, 2019). Data from the 1997–2000 Medical Expenditure Panel Survey revealed lower diagnosis and treatment of ADHD children among minority youth (Stevens et al., 2005). What are the implications of the under treatment of ADHD in this vulnerable population?

IMPLICATIONS OF UNDERDIAGNOSIS OF ADHD

Untreated ADHD is associated with lowered self-esteem and poor social function outcomes, as shown in a systematic review of 127 studies (Harpin et al., 2016). Similarly, in a meta-analysis of 351 studies from multiple countries, long-term outcomes for participants with untreated ADHD included elevated risk of drug use/addictive behavior, academic failure, and antisocial behavior (Shaw et al., 2010). Thus, minority youth with ADHD are at extreme risk due to the lack of effective intervention. What can clinicians do to address this significant issue?

CLINICAL INTERVENTION

As noted above, clinicians need to adopt cultural sensitivity and take socioeconomic factors into account while evaluating children from multicultural families. Whenever possible, patients should be evaluated and treated by clinicians of the same background to render services that enhance the level of care. Further, healthcare providers should practice psychoeducation with the family in explaining how they reached their diagnosis and the risks and benefits of treatment. Many minority parents who are bringing their children into treatment say that their own parents would never have brought them as children into treatment. In other words, there is a cultural gap regarding mental health and services that these parents are trying to bridge between their own parents (from the "old country") and their "American" children. When intervention is so foreign to the family, they require significant parent training to understand the diagnosis and facilitate effective treatment (Alvarado & Modsto-Lowe, 2017). Providing resources to the parents, such as books (e.g., Hallowell & Ratey, 2021) and referrals to advocacy organizations (e.g., CHADD; Children and Adults with Attention Deficit Hyperactivity Disorder) can be invaluable to help them understand the disorder. Below is a case example that illustrates the importance of sensitivity to cultural values surrounding ADHD and the positive impact of parent training.

Joshua, an exuberant, 8-year-old African American boy was referred for therapy due to concerns about poor impulse control, low frustration tolerance and aggressive outbursts. His parents were very distressed about his behaviors and categorized him as "bad" and "rude." His father was particularly concerned about his aggression and tended to be punitive and retaliatory. Joshua was diagnosed with attention deficit disorder, but the parents did not want to put him on medication, preferring to intervene behaviorally and therapeutically. During parent counseling sessions, I provided psychoeducation about attention deficit disorder, explaining how Joshua's symptoms were directly related to his brain "wiring." We then collaboratively brainstormed about techniques to help him contain his impulses. I was careful to remain sensitive to the parents' cultural values and reframed their attempts to discipline Joshua as their commitment to Joshua's socialization and education. After several months of sessions, Joshua's father tearfully exclaimed that he thinks he has ADD as well and that he was feeling very guilty and ashamed of his past harshness to Joshua. Joshua's behaviors improved but he continued to have difficulty focusing during class. Two years after his diagnosis, his parents elected to try a psychopharmacological treatment. We remained in contact over this time period and parents reported that Joshua was doing well academically and socially.

LEARNING DISORDERS

Prevalence

Similar to ADHD, there are wide disparities in disability identification by race and ethnicity. However, the statistics on Learning Disorders reflect a very different pattern than ADHD. Whereas students of color are underrepresented in children diagnosed with attention disorders, they are over-represented among children diagnosed with learning disabilities. Based on a demographic study that encompasses the six million students with disabilities that receive services, black students are 40 percent more likely and American Indians 70 percent more likely to be diagnosed with learning disorders (Harper, 2017). There are many factors that contribute to the disproportionately large number of black children in special education placements, including trauma, stress, lack of parent education, nutritional deficiencies, and unstable learning environments that can all impact cognitive development (Bigelow, 2006; Saifi & Mehmood, 2011; De Bellis & Zisk, 2014). There is also the problem of biased diagnosis, with children being diagnosed with learning disorders inappropriately. In fact, black youth are 2.5 times more likely to be diagnosed as compared with white children—although in metro areas within states such as Florida, North Carolina, and Connecticut, minority children have the same or lower learning disability rates as compared with non-minority children (Coutinho et al. 2002). Let us consider the causes of this disparity.

SOCIOECONOMIC STATUS

Disproportionate identification of students with a learning disability occurs among groups who are already socially disadvantaged (Deshler et al., 2004). The causes for this are complex. Firstly, higher prevalence of learning disorders among minority children has been linked to high levels of maternal and social deprivation (Emerson, 1997). Children from disadvantaged backgrounds do not have the same resources as majority and higher income children, to the detriment of their cognitive development. Previous research confirms that resources in the home during early childhood is strongly correlated with the development of both cognitive and learning ability (Shonkoff & Phillips, 2000). In fact, black males who are born to mothers who have poor educational background are most at risk for being diagnosed with learning disorders and placed in special education settings (Ramey et al., 1978). Thus, identification of learning problems may also reflect social differences as well as learning differences (Fernando, 1989).

Whether such challenges constitute actual learning disabilities is questionable. Some children's learning disabilities have been identified as "sociocultural" or "reversible," as their deficits seem primarily due to socioeconomic status and/or cultural factors rather than inborn anatomical differences. In other words, with appropriate support and enrichment, their cognitive skills will improve. Of course, there are some deficits that are due to environmental factors that cannot be reversed, particularly when they are very severe.

Lower socio-economic status and its associated stresses may have a direct impact on the brain, however, through epigenetic processes (Raizada & Kishiyama, 2010). Epigenetic effects can markedly change a phenotype (behavioral or physical expression of genetic inheritance); epigenetic changes can be caused by experiences, such as exposure to environmental toxins, changes in dietary health, or major stressful events. These experiences, in other words, can make permanent changes in what genes are turned off or on, creating lasting alterations in how the body (and thus, brain and behavior) operate. Moreover, epigenetic changes can be transmitted across mammalian generations, meaning that what the mother experiences during pregnancy can influence the behavior of her daughter and granddaughter via changes in gene expression. Thus, this research may pave the way to intervention during pregnancy or early infancy (Nigg, 2012; Schaen, 2006).

INAPPROPRIATE DIAGNOSIS AND ASSESSMENTS

Poor and inappropriate diagnostic procedures and/or discrimination may also play a role in the disproportionate identification of certain students (Shifrer et al., 2011). The Educational Longitudinal Study of 2002 described national patterns in learning disability identification that highlighted the association between socioeconomic status and identification (Shifrer et al., 2011), suggesting children with less financial resources may be more likely to be erroneously classified as having LDs. The cultural bias of IQ testing is well recognized, although efforts have been made to administer the test in a culturally sensitive manner (Fernando, 1989). We also need to be alert to clinician bias and the tendency to misinterpret certain behaviors that are more reflective of cultural norms rather than pathology. For example, a child who is guarded and defensive during the assessment and does not put forth his or her best effort may be uncomfortable due to the cultural barrier between the child and the clinician. His or her test results need to be interpreted with that variable in mind and to understand that the child may underperform in that setting.

SPECIAL EDUCATION AS CULTURAL/SOCIAL BIAS

Some researchers have suggested that placement in special education is a form of racial bias (Reid & Knight, 2006). As black children are over-represented in segregated special education classes, they suffer from both discrimination due to the stigma of not being mainstreamed, and from diagnosis of learning disorders—placing them in double jeopardy regarding ability to succeed both academically and professionally (Artiles, 2021). Thus, identification of learning problems may also reflect social differences as well as learning differences (Fernando, 1989). Further, the special education placements are not necessarily an adequate intervention for these children's academic challenges. In my own experience, working in the New York City public schools, I have certainly seen a large number of black and Hispanic children in special education placements that are grossly inadequate and are not customized to the child's individualized learning profile. In this case, it is not the placement of children in special education, per se, that is discriminating—but the poor quality of the special education provided.

BILINGUALISM

Bilingualism is another significant variable in the diagnosis of learning disabilities. There is a disproportionate representation of language minorities in children diagnosed with learning disorders. Further, immigrant parents who are often non-native speakers can encounter significant challenges advocating for their children's needs in an often-overwhelming system. With current diagnostic methods, it can be difficult to distinguish between a lack of English language proficiency and a learning disability (Klingner & Harry, 2006).

Clearly, bilingualism can interfere with test results, and it is preferable for children to be assessed in their first language. A recent survey of psychologists revealed that many lacked the cultural sensitivity and training that would be optimal to conduct assessment and feedback (Mindt et al., 2008). As mentioned earlier, it is important to assess the child in his or her primary language. With so few psychologists able to test in languages other than English, however, use of an interpreter is often necessary. Interpreting by family members should be avoided due to potential conflict within the family (Farooq & Fear, 2003). Working with professional interpreters also brings challenges. When negotiating the interpreter-clinician relationship, good practice entails ensuring the interpreter is well versed in the information needed, agrees to a collaborative model, ensures that the translation reflects cultural context and affirms the importance of confidentiality (Nadirshaw, 1997). Below I present an example of a testing that was compromised by lack of attention to and understanding of cultural and linguistic issues.

An assessment of a 7-year-old bilingual (Spanish) girl revealed learning and attention difficulties that were confirmed by a teacher report and classroom observation. The verbal feedback to the parents appeared to go well, and they seemed to agree with the results and recommendations. However, upon receipt of the report, the mother emailed a detailed letter contesting the results and questioning the rapport the child had with the tester. She commented that, although her daughter may have appeared cooperative and willing, she had not been performing optimally in school or during the test situation. She further contended that the testing and results were invalid based on the daughter's inadequate English-language skills.

Upon my second meeting with the parents, I acknowledged the mother's email and asked for feedback from the parents regarding the testing information. We reviewed the areas of discrepancy between the parents' perspectives and the test data. For example, the parents perceived the child as being more academically and intellectually capable than her scores reflected. I offered to further assess the child's language skills, as the mother felt that the child's scores were deflated due to her child's bilingualism. Although the initial testing contained some language assessments, I offered to augment these tests with some more nuanced tests of language ability. The mother was enthusiastic about getting more information and was relieved that I took her comments seriously. It became clear that the child felt most comfortable in a bilingual environment and was underperforming in school and during the testing due to the different cultural and linguistic expectations.

CULTURAL COMPETENCE GUIDELINES

The organization Ethnicity and Equality created guidelines on how to engage people with learning disabilities from black and minority ethnic communities in a culturally sensitive manner (Ethnicity and Equality: Foundation for people with Learning Disabilities, 2009). They suggest that the practitioner understand his or her own biases, be committed to celebrating rather than denigrating cultural differences, and provide culturally competent assessment, communication, and care. Similarly, being aware of the income level, educational level, housing status, and overall health of family members is important when practitioners are planning services for people with learning disabilities. For example, after school support may not be readily available or affordable for lower income families.

It is important for clinicians to understand that many beliefs and worldviews of minority families diverge from the majority perspective, for example the emphasis on eye contact, verbal expressiveness, and punctuality (Sue & Sue, 1999). Some cultures believe that direct eye contact is rude. The concept of time may differ across cultures and patterns of emotional expression can vary widely across cultures. Some cultures are quite restricted in emotional expression and other cultures are the opposite. These differences need to be recognized when working with people from ethnic/minority communities and intervention and assessment techniques should be modified as necessary. Of note, while these recommended best practices are provided by an organization focused specifically upon learning disabilities, they are equally applicable to all culturally diverse individuals with neurocognitive challenges.

AUTISM SPECTRUM DISORDER

I will now discuss the factors of race, culture, and socioeconomic status in the assessment and intervention with patients with autism spectrum disorder.

Prevalence

Autism awareness and access to services are increasing, both in general and across racial and ethnic groups. In fact, the prevalence of autism spectrum disorder diagnoses rose between 2018 and 2020, continuing a long running trend (CDC, 2020). In 2020, an estimated one in 36 8-year-olds was diagnosed with autism, up from one in 44 in 2018. The prevalence was roughly four percent in boys and one percent in girls.

In the past decade, differences have been documented regarding diagnosis of ASD. In 2020, the prevalence among minority children still lagged behind that of white children. At that time, white children were about 19 percent more likely than black children and 65 percent more likely than Hispanic children to be diagnosed with autism. For example, a study of 406 Medicaid-eligible children revealed that white children received diagnoses of autism spectrum disorder at 6.3 years old, whereas black children were diagnosed later, at 7.9 years (Mandell et al., 2002). The discrepancy in parent awareness was illustrated in a study that interviewed parents of toddlers with autism spectrum disorder (Mandell et al., 2007). They found that black parents reported significantly fewer autism concerns and fewer concerns about socially restricted and repetitive behavior as compared with white parents. In fact, black children were nearly twice as likely to be misdiagnosed with conduct disorders prior to an ASD diagnosis, which the authors speculated was possibly due to the way the parents reported symptoms to healthcare providers (Mandell et al., 2007). Consistent with the findings mentioned previously, other U.S. cohort studies have shown that the black community and people with a lower socioeconomic status have lower ASD rates (Durkin et al., 2010).

As advanced paternal age is associated with an increase in autism risk, and fathers of white children tend to be older than those of black or Hispanic children, paternal age may be a risk factor (Furfaro, 2017). Further, cultural and linguistic diversity influence the identification of students with ASD, with underrepresentation of diverse students (Tincani et al., 2009). These differences were attributed to a combination of clinician prejudice, unequal access to healthcare, and lack of parental information and awareness about autism (Donohue et al., 2017).

However, more recent studies suggest this pattern may be changing. Recent CDC reports indicated that autism diagnoses are now more prevalent among 8-year-old black children as compared with white children (Anthes, 2023). Further, a recent cross-sectional study using nationally representative data for 2014 through 2019 of over half a million individuals showed black individuals to surpass white individuals regarding diagnosis of ASD, particularly at a younger age (Yuan et al., 2021). Similarly, an ASD prevalence cohort study of over seven million students in England found that the national prevalence was 1.76 percent, with the highest prevalence in black students and the lowest in Roma/Irish children. Moreover, children from lower socioeconomic backgrounds were more frequently diagnosed with ASD (Roman-Urrestarazu et al., 2021). These findings are in line with a population study in the United States that found higher ASD rates in immigrants with foreign-born mothers (Becerra et al., 2014). This pattern might indicate improved screening, awareness, and access to service among underserved groups. Specifically, the rise in prevalence among black children may be partially due to improved access to health care in recent years. Of course, there is also the risk that sociodemographic differences may lead to overdiagnosis of ASD in nonwhite and lower SES groups, as found with ADHD.

These discrepant findings and the questions they raise highlight the need for more standardized assessments of autism spectrum disorder and further investigation into the possible impact of race, culture, and socioeconomic status on diagnosis. It could be that white children are truly more likely to have ASD due to the older age of white fathers. Concomitantly, the traditional under diagnosis of black children could be due to their families' lack of information about ASD or clinicians who perceive black children as aggressive, and conduct disordered rather than agitated due to their ASD. Future research will have to disentangle these complex threads.

Autism diagnoses also vary according to gender; in 2012, the Centers for Disease Control and Prevention estimated that boys were 4.7 times as likely as girls to receive an autism diagnosis (Centers for Disease Control and Prevention, 2023). By 2018, the ratio dipped to 4.2 to one (Centers for Disease Control and Prevention, 2023). And, in data released in 2023, the figure was 3.8 to one (Centers for Disease Control and Prevention, 2023). In that new analysis, the autism rate of girls surpassed one percent, the highest ever recorded. Older women are also being diagnosed with autism due to more sophisticated and nuanced methods of assessment and the recognition that girls with autism present differently than boys. Girls tend to camouflage their social challenges more successfully. They also tend to develop anxiety and depression more often. These characteristics can obscure the underlying autism and lead to misdiagnosis. It should be noted that girls and boys in general display different behavioral characteristics, such as better linguistic and social skills (Lai et al., 2015). This likely impacts the expression of autism symptoms across the genders.

Bias in Assessment

As noted above, the varied findings about differential prevalence across racial and other demographic groups have been attributed in part to bias in assessment. As such, research into possible assessment bias is important. The Autism Diagnostic Observation Schedule (Lord et al., 2012) is now regarded as the reference standard assessment for ASD. Despite multiple studies demonstrating its utility and accuracy, there have been only a few studies examining the instrument for racial bias. Item-level bias was found in a small study, that is, holding level of overall behavioral symptoms constant, three items were answered differently due to race and ethnicity (Harrison et al., 2017). A large study of over six thousand children found low bias overall, although 11 percent of the diagnostic items demonstrated bias and the magnitude of bias was moderate-to-large for only two repetitive/restricted behavior interest items. These results suggest that further research is needed to address some evidence of under-detection of ASD symptoms in black/African American children (Kalb et al., 2022). Assessment bias and under-diagnosis can also lead to significant differences in intervention and use of services. I will now discuss the discrepancies in service use among different ethnic and socioeconomic groups.

Disparities in Service Use

A comprehensive review of research on racial, ethnic, and socioeconomic disparities in autism diagnoses revealed that treatment disparities exist for access to care, referral frequency, number of service hours, and proportion of unmet service needs. Several studies revealed that African American families and those from low-income households reported lower quality of care (Smith et al., 2020). As proper early intervention can be a crucial factor in improving the quality of life for children with autism, this discrepancy in services is a significant issue in long term functional outcome (Grabovschi et al., 2013). Early Intervention typically consists of intense, one on one sessions with the child using Applied Behavior Analysis to help shape appropriate behaviors. In addition, children receive speech therapy, physical therapy, occupational therapy and educational services. These services can greatly facilitate language and social development in children with ASD.

Such comprehensive services, however, can be lacking in communities with minority and lower income families as they tend to be under-resourced. One promising solution is to deliver low-cost, intensive behavioral intervention through organizations already active within the broader community, making these resources more accessible and affordable. One such program developed by the Michigan Early Learning Institute has provided early intensive behavioral intervention in community settings (such as Headstart programs), with an emphasis on serving children and families on Medicaid. This program focused on providing early intervention by providers who were trained in the principles of applied behavior analysis (ABA) along with parent training and participation, that is, teaching the parents how to parent more effectively using ABA (Plavnick et al., 2020). As these interventions have shown to be effective with children with autism, access to such programs for low SES families is essential for their children's healthy development (Reichow, 2011).

Cultural Differences in Working with Autistic Individuals and Their Families

When autistic individuals and their families from non-majority groups do access care, clinicians' insensitivity to cultural differences can impede the effectiveness of that care. The below case example illustrates the importance of exploring cultural beliefs when working with parents of children with autism.

An adult woman who was an immigrant from East Asia was referred for treatment due to depression and anxiety. Clinical interview revealed that her depression began when her second son was diagnosed with autism and began to receive intensive early intervention services. The mother had difficulty engaging with her son although she loved him and wanted to connect. She described feeling disconnected from him and not knowing how to engage. The child demonstrated perseverative, repetitive behaviors, such as playing obsessively with action figures. In addition, he had difficulty falling asleep, was nonverbal and would often cry, yell, run away, and engage in aggressive behaviors. These behaviors frightened the mother, and she began to withdraw from her son. After several months of treatment, she revealed that she believed her son was possessed by an evil spirit and she was scared of him. The therapist worked with these beliefs and was able to help her to better understand her son's condition. She began to participate in his care and learned from his therapists how to intervene more effectively when he was demonstrating aggressive behaviors.

Culture is also relevant when addressing the social skills deficits so central to autism. For example, lowering your eyes when spoken to can be a culturally encouraged behavior that might be misidentified as poor eye contact. Similarly, Western values emphasize being assertive and being an individual whereas other cultures are more focused on deference to group norms. In a review of the literature on social skills training in the United States for individuals with autism, Davenport et al. (2018) found that only five studies incorporated cultural adaptations to the interventions and that minority populations were underrepresented in the study samples. Thus, careful consideration should be given to the cultural values and identity particularly of ethnic/minority groups when facilitating social skills. In fact, being neurodivergent in itself is seen by many patients as an essential part of their culture and identity. I will now discuss this burgeoning movement to embrace neurodiversity and claim it as part of one's cultural identity.

EMBRACING NEURODIVERSITY

There is a current movement that advocates neurodivergent people to embrace their neurodivergence as part of their identity. There is a distinct community and cultural aspect to this phenomenon that is largely focused on people with autism but also extends to other people with neurocognitive impairments.

As awareness of neurocognitive impairments has become more widespread, there is a burgeoning movement to embrace differences and celebrate neurodiversity. Particularly, young adults with autism are creating a community, organizing clubs on campus, developing safe spaces for socializing, and advocating for themselves. This movement resembles other civil rights movements to gain equal rights and empower a marginalized community. Advocating for accommodations and modifications in school and in the workspace is part of this important movement. Using the internet to socialize with like-minded individuals who also identify as neurodivergent is an essential aspect of socialization for these individuals with ASD. They often share common obsessive interests in niche pursuits, such as certain movies, books, TV series or video games. They meet online and may never meet in person but nonetheless consider themselves part of a rich and varied community. Books such as *The Power of Neurodiversity* (Armstrong, 2011) and organizations such as Autism Speaks are resources that provide support and a blueprint for this perspective. The following case example illustrates the significance of these connections to a patient with ASD.

Eugene, a young adult with autism (mentioned in earlier chapters) introduced the session by stating, "I have had a tough week but also had a very good thing happen to me." He then showed me that he had received a care package from an online friend who knew that he had been struggling. The friend had sent him several beautiful homemade books and posters that were focused on their mutual interests. He explained that he met the friend online and that they exchange gifts as a way of cheering each other up. These interactions are very meaningful to Eugene and help him feel supported as well as socially connected.

CONCLUSION

When working with individuals with neurocognitive challenges from ethnic/minority groups, it is critical to take cultural factors into account. There are significant discrepancies in the prevalence of neurocognitive disorders among ethnic/minority groups, which appear to be multiply determined, reflecting differential access to assessment and treatment as well as possible over- or under-diagnosis from clinician bias. Clinicians need to be sensitive to the issues of bilingualism, unequal access to healthcare, and the impact of parental cultural values in the family's perception or understanding of the child's condition and the treatments available. In addition, cultural competence requires attunement to the patient's cultural values, particularly when intervening with social skills.

Chapter Ten

Future Directions

It has been the aim of this book to convey the powerful and pervasive psychological challenges that individuals with neurocognitive disorders face. Throughout the book, we addressed effective methods of assessment and treatment with these patients given the complexity and far-reaching impact of their disorders. First, we discussed how to diagnose neurocognitive disorders using a broad range of assessment tools. We next explored the impact of assessment and provided specific recommendations on how to use the test results most effectively in treatment. We then reviewed the use of accommodations and modifications, and the emotional effect of these interventions on patients.

The optimal approach to intervention with these patients requires multiple foci: patients' neurocognitive deficits, the psychiatric symptoms that accompany these challenges, and the traumatic aspects of the patients' development due to their neurocognitive challenges and other people's responses to them (i.e., parents, peers, and teachers). A complex and nuanced treatment approach is proposed, one that includes psychoeducation and problem solving—helping the patients understand the neurocognitive underpinnings of their challenges, dispelling misconceptions about their learning disabilities, and devising effective strategies for their day-to-day difficulties.

This book also addressed special topics such as transference/countertransference when working with patients with neurocognitive disorders. Given patients' deeply shameful feelings about their deficits, such feelings of shame often surface in the treatment when these deficits are addressed or exposed. Patients' defensive responses to these painful emotions can lead to difficult transference/countertransference enactments, which may challenge the clinician's comfort level. Likewise, therapists must be prepared to negotiate patients' intense feelings of guilt, frustration, and the desire for autonomy. For clinicians with their own learning challenges, the use of self-disclosure can be a powerful tool to dispel shame and provide a positive role model for patients. We also discussed the specific impact of the COVID-19 pandemic on children, adolescents, and adults with neurocognitive impairment. Nonetheless, despite the pandemic's pointed impact on mental health, some children and adolescents were actually able to thrive and even demonstrated improvements in their social and emotional functioning (Chawla et al., 2021; Silk et al., 2022).

It is critical to consider these issues within the context of culture and ethnicity, however, as there are significant discrepancies in the diagnosis and assessment of neurocognitive disorders across ethnic/minority groups. Effective intervention across diverse populations requires sensitivity to the issues of bilingualism, unequal access to healthcare, and the impact of parental cultural values in the family's ability to obtain services for the child. In addition, it is important to be aware of the patient's cultural values, particularly when intervening with social skills.

FUTURE DIRECTIONS IN RESEARCH

Neurobiology

There has been promising research into the neurobiological substrates and etiology of neurocognitive disorders—but additional research is needed for a full understanding of these syndromes. Elucidation of genetic processes can shed light on the development of such disorders. This research is strongest for ADHD, as a meta-analysis identified several genetic markers associated with this disorder (Gizer et al., 2009). In addition, functional and structural neuroimaging studies have identified alterations in the frontal lobe in ADHD, adding to our understanding of its neurobiology (Bush, 2011). Similarly, there have been significant advances in the study of the neurobiology and genetics of ASD as well as in early identification and intervention techniques (Parallada et al., 2014; Johnson & Meyers, 2007). Further, although neuroimaging studies of NVLD are few, this research method offers promise to further elucidate the etiology and underlying mechanisms, information which can potentially guide intervention (Katz, et al., 2001).

Promising directions in intervention with ASD patients include recognition of the common psychiatric comorbidities, new medications to treat symptoms, and enhanced intervention with adults with ASD (Damiano et al., 2014; Matson et al., 2013). As of yet, there is no established protocol for relating specific child, family, target behavior, and treatment variables to individualized treatment regimens based on the neurobiology of the patient (Schreibman, 2000). In this vein, precision medicine may provide a promising development for the treatment of ASD, particularly to address subgroups with associated difficulties, such as ADHD, irritability/aggression, and sleep difficulties (Anagnostou, 2018). Precision medicine is medical care designed to optimize efficiency or therapeutic benefits for particular groups of patients, especially by using genetic or molecular profiling. It is an emerging approach for disease treatment and prevention that takes in account individual variability in genes, environment, and lifestyle for each person.

USE OF COMPUTER TECHNOLOGY

The use of computerized technology is a burgeoning area that has had a wide impact on individuals with neurocognitive disorders, offering significant promise but also drawbacks. Future research is critical to clarify both the benefits and risks of this rapidly developing technology.

Use of technology has been proposed as a revolutionary breakthrough in working with patients with ADD (More et al., 2008) and ASD (Jiminez-Munoz et al., 2022). Software can provide step-by-step instruction, wait for responses, offer immediate feedback, and allow students to work at their own pace. It is thought that these experiences facilitate learning in students who are typically inattentive; they empower the students to be actively involved in the lesson and increase their motivation and confidence (Fitzgerald, 1994). Indeed, use of computer programs has led to documented improvements in the areas of parent training and social skills for children with ADHD (Xie et al., 2013; More, 2008; Margalit, 1995). However, Xu (2002) reviewed empirical studies that assessed the efficacy of technology as a tool for students with ADHD, and they identified methodological difficulties with the studies demonstrating the efficacy of computer-based instruction and computer assisted cognitive training and concluded that there is no firm evidence supporting the use of computer-assisted instruction and training with children with ADD. Computerized assessment of ADHD was also found to have limited value and needed to be considered in conjunction with other findings. Thus, there is need for research with greater methodological rigor in this fast-growing domain.

Video game technology has been shown to positively impact people with dyslexia and improve reading skills. A small study of dyslexic children found that video games that are targeted to improve attention also improved reading speed and accuracy, which has been attributed to improvements in visual attention, an area of deficit for children with dyslexia (Franceschini et al., 2017). As people with developmental dyslexia show difficulties in several perceptual modalities (Vidyasagar et al., 2010), these programs are specifically targeted to improve visual skills (Francheshini et al., 2013). A recent meta-analysis shows that video games led to improved information processing in both quasi-experimental and true experiment studies (Green & Bavelier, 2003). It must be stressed, however, that only specific video games that target attention and visual processing are useful in increasing reading abilities.

Further, use of technologies, such as speech-to-text, have revolutionized the ability of neurodivergent learners to write. Examples of these technologies include dictation into the computer; spellcheck, which provides feedback about misspelled words and offers alternative spellings; and Grammarly, which provides the same service with grammar and syntax.

In sum, the data suggests significant benefit from these technologies for individuals with learning disabilities. Integration of computer programs into classrooms is a complex and cost-intensive proposition, however. Teachers need to be trained in the specific use of these technologies so they can use them effectively in the classroom. Students require access to the programs and the computers to run them. Likewise, a survey study of the current use of computer integration in preschool special education indicated that teachers desire more training and technical assistance in the adoption of computer technology into the classroom and ask that the software better reflect the developmental needs of children with disabilities (Judge, 2000). The survey also showed that teachers primarily use computer technology to develop and reinforce academic skills. Thus, the use of technology is a promising area of intervention but requires additional rigorous research for maximal efficacy and successful implementation.

PSYCHOSOCIAL INTERVENTIONS

Psychosocial treatments, such as academic and interpersonal skills training, target various areas of difficulty, including time management, organization, planning and self-esteem. These treatments also provide psychoeducation about symptoms, introduce new coping repertoires, and support individuals' strengths (Hill et al., 2000; Schultz et al., 2017; Ratey et al., 1992).

Psychosocial programs to improve social and emotional functioning among students with learning disorders have proven to be effective with college students (Manganello, 1992). The author identified multiple causes of psychosocial problems among LD students: pragmatic language deficits, social skills deficits (i.e., misreading social cues) and sequelae of NVLD (including deficits in adapting to new situations), poor social judgment, and misunderstanding of humor. As these deficits are multi-determined, in order to be effective, a multidisciplinary approach involving learning specialists, mental health professionals and educators, is recommended. In addition, education about substance abuse and career counseling services are valuable adjunct services as students with LD and ADHD are vulnerable to substance abuse (Fox & Forbing, 1991).

Initially, research on psychosocial treatments for adults with ADHD could be summarized as "entirely anecdotal" (1996 Child and Adolescent Psychiatric Diplomates, 1997). Currently, there is a growing literature documenting the efficacy of psychosocial treatments such as behavioral parent training, behavioral classroom management, and peer-focused behavioral interventions (Schultz et al., 2017; Pelham et al., 1998). However, there was great variability across the studies regarding the methods of ADD diagnosis and the instruments used to measure improvement. In addition, sample sizes were generally small, there were few randomized trials, and sparse long-term follow-up studies exist. Rigorous empirical studies are recommended to assess efficacy and improve psychosocial services, such as skills training, group therapy and intervention with families to address the common behaviors associated with ADD, including impulsivity, low frustration tolerance, and rigidity, that contribute to significant social and behavioral problems at home and in the classroom (Ramsay, J. R., & Rostain, A. L., 2007).

Over the past several decades, a plethora of school-based interventions for students with ADHD have been studied. Yet there are considerable limitations to this research (Dupaul et al., 2009; Klingner et al., 2003). Dupaul et al. (2009) identified that outcome studies must go beyond a focus on simply reducing ADHD symptoms, such as impulsivity and poor focus, as children with ADD demonstrate extensive deficits across multiple areas of functioning. In addition, these interventions, which typically consist of behavioral interventions and academic strategies, vary according to the resources of the school, the complexity of the intervention, the teachers' readiness to intervene, and the match between teaching style and intervention (Klingner et al., 2003).

With regard to patients with ASD, there is tremendous need for intervention to address the social deficits that are a hallmark of this disorder. A significant area of challenge for patients with ASD is effective implementation of psychosocial techniques, and further research thus is indicated to improve efficacy and delivery of these interventions.

In sum, psychosocial treatments are another potentially effective method of intervention that requires further research regarding implementation and outcomes.

NEUROFEEDBACK AND MINDFULNESS

Biofeedback has also been suggested as an intervention for students with ADHD. In a review by Xu (2002), it was suggested that biofeedback might serve as a useful ancillary treatment—but it could not be recommended as a primary treatment due to time, cost, and the lack of randomized, double-blind studies with placebo-control conditions (Xu, 2002). In addition, mindfulness meditation training in ADHD has been shown to improve attention, reduce stress, and improve mood (Mitchell et al., 2015; Zylowska et al., 2007). However, a systematic review of mindfulness training for individuals (children, adolescents, and adults) with ADHD concluded that it is unclear whether this intervention is effective due to the small number of studies available and the limitations of study design in the reviewed studies. Future research is required to conclude whether to offer mindfulness as a primary treatment for ADHD.

INCLUSION

The inclusion of special needs students into the mainstream is another area that has received attention as a future trend in education. Research has shown that including special education students in mainstream classes facilitates academic achievement, improved social functioning and better appreciation of neurocognitive disorders (Kurth & Mastergeorge, 2010). Nonetheless, we need to further study how to implement inclusion effectively (Putnam et al., 1995). In a survey of 37 educators, study participants indicated awareness of this trend and also expressed concern about how to implement inclusion in their classroom (Putnam et al., 1995). The future model for inclusion is a multi-dimensional approach where educational placement is tailored for the individual's specific needs and there is a continuum from special education schools to inclusion in the mainstream (Norwich, 2008). Likewise, Armstrong (2012) offers a comprehensive model of strength-based strategies in the classroom to help students with special needs. He emphasizes accentuating the positive and using technology, environmental modifications, and social resources, such as peers and support staff. (Armstrong, 2012). These techniques need to be more extensively studied and implemented so we develop best practices in how to include these students in the mainstream as much as possible.

In sum, assessment and intervention with individuals with neurocognitive challenges is a complicated and nuanced process that entails devising an individualized profile of the individuals' strengths and challenges, addressing the emotional sequelae that is concomitant with the disorder, and helping the individual celebrate his or her areas of strength academically, socially, and professionally. As neurocognitive disorders have a far-reaching impact on individuals and their families, it is essential that clinicians become well versed regarding the most common disorders and associated psychosocial sequelae so that they can offer effective treatment to their patients.

Appendix

Neuropsychological Evaluation

Name: Moira
Date of Birth: xx/xx/xxxx
Age: 11 years 0 months
Grade: 5

Date of Testing: xx/xx/xx, xx/xx/xx, xx/xx/xx
Date of Report: xx/xx/xx
Examiner: Jane Doe, Ed.M., NCSP
Supervisor: Nechama Sorscher, Ph.D.

REASON FOR REFERRAL

Moira is an 11-year-old girl who was referred for an initial neuropsychological evaluation at the recommendation of Dr. Jane Doe. This consultation is subsequent to recent evaluations in which Moira has been diagnosed with an auditory processing disorder (Dr. Doe, xx/xx/xx) and possible anxiety, depressive, learning, language and attention disorders (Dr. Doe, xx/xx/xx). Parent and teacher reports indicate that Moira mishears, needs repetition and has trouble following directions. In addition, Moira is distracted by noisy environments, finds it difficult to focus when background noise is present and is disorganized. She appears aware of her challenges and, as her parents report, she often comments on her skills in a self-deprecating manner. Thus, a cognitive, academic and personality evaluation was conducted to assess Moira's current level of functioning and to provide recommendations for intervention.

Background Information

Background information has been redacted for client privacy.

Behavioral Observations

Moira presents as a sweet, well mannered, and socially engaging young girl who was consistently friendly and cooperative throughout testing. She appeared to be comfortable upon meeting the examiner as well as with the testing environment. She arrived with her mother for all her sessions. Moira went willingly into the assessment room. Rapport was easily established with the examiner. She maintained good eye contact. Moira demonstrated difficulty processing auditory information, as she often asked the examiner to repeat and clarify instructions. Moreover, Moira needed repetition and prompting to converse. She often asked, "What?" "Wait what?" and "Huh?" She admitted to having trouble remembering with statements like, "I don't remember what it is called," and "I forget." In many cases, and where allowed, the stimulus question had to be repeated more than once for a response. She did mishear in a one-to-one situation. She was slow to respond and needed more time to formulate her answers.

Moira evidenced a remarkable work ethic as she sat up straight in her chair and completed all that was asked of her. She was consistently invested in producing her best work, and would take time as was necessary to finish problems. She tended to utilize almost all or more than the allotted time per task. Fine-motor tasks appeared significantly taxing on Moira. More specifically, her approach to pencil-and-paper activities was slow, careful and methodical as she reviewed every mark before advancing to further items. Such tasks required extended time and sustained effort. In addition, she demonstrated a pressured grip on the pencil, resulting in dark pencil marks and laborious writing. Moira complained of hand fatigue and was observed shaking her hand for relief.

Overall, Moira was highly motivated and demonstrated a genuine concern for her performance. She was cooperative throughout testing and took an active role as a participant by asking questions and sharing information. Difficulties with auditory processing, word-retrieval, and fine-motor tasks were observed. Given Moira's overall effort, the present test results provide a valid and accurate assessment of her current level of functioning.

TESTS ADMINISTERED

General Intelligence

Wechsler Intelligence Scale for Children—Fifth Edition (WISC-V)

Academic Ability

Gray-Oral Reading Tests—Fifth Edition (GORT-5)
Test of Written Language—Third Edition (TOWL-3), select
Wechsler Individual Achievement Test—Third Edition (WIAT-III), select
Woodcock Johnson Tests of Achievement—Fourth Edition, Form A (WJ-IV), select

Learning/Memory

Wide Range Assessment of Memory and Learning—Second Edition (WRAML2)

Auditory Processing

A Test for Auditory Processing Disorder in Children (SCAN-C)

Attention/Executive Functioning

Conners Continuous Performance Test—Third Edition (CPT-3)
Wisconsin Card Sorting Test (WCST)

Visuomotor

Beery-Bukentika Developmental Test of Visual Motor Integration—Sixth Edition (Beery VMI)

Personality

Behavior Assessment System for Children—2nd Edition Parent Rating Scales (BASC-2 PRS)
Behavior Assessment System for Children—2nd Edition Teacher Rating Scales (BASC-2 TRS)
Rorschach Inkblot Test
Thematic Apperception Test (TAT)

Results: General Intelligence/Cognitive

Wechsler Intelligence Scale for Children—Fourth Edition (WISC-V)

Composite	*SS*	*Percentile*	*Qualitative*
Full Scale IQ (FSIQ)	95	37	Average
Verbal Comprehension Index (VCI)	98	45	Average
Visual Spatial Index (VSI)	94	34	Average
Fluid Reasoning Index (FRI)	109	73	Average
Working Memory Index (WMI)	88	21	Low Average
Processing Speed Index (PSI)	80	9	Low Average

Verbal Comprehension	**SS***
Similarities	9
Vocabulary	10
Visual Spatial	**SS***
Block Design	7
Visual Puzzles	11
Fluid Reasoning	**SS***
Figure Weights	11
Matrix Reasoning	12
Working Memory	**SS***
Picture Span	8
Digit Span	8
Processing Speed	**SS***
Coding	8
Symbol Search	5

* >16=Very Superior; 15–14 = Superior; 13–12 = High Average; 11–8 = Average; 7 = Low Average; <7 = Below Average

Index Comparisons	*Difference*	*Significant*
VCI—PSI	18	Y

The Wechsler Intelligence Scale for Children–Fifth Edition (WISC-V) was used to assess Moira's cognitive functioning. The Full-Scale IQ (FSIQ) is derived from a combination of the ten primary subtest scores and is considered to be the most representative estimation of a child's cognitive ability. According to the FSIQ, Moira's general cognitive ability is within the Average range and falls in the 37th percentile, suggesting that her overall thinking and reasoning abilities equal or exceed those of approximately 37 percent of similarly aged children (FSIQ=95). There was significant score variability between the core cognitive areas that were assessed by the WISC-V (i.e., her verbal comprehension, visual spatial and fluid reasoning scores were much higher than her working memory and processing speed scores); therefore, the FSIQ should be interpreted with caution. Moira presents with variability between her verbal and nonverbal abilities that is consistent with a DSM-5 diagnosis of Unspecified Neurodevelopmental Disorder (315.9). The pattern of her subtest scores underscores Moira's adequate verbal, visual-spatial and fluid reasoning skills, while also revealing the extent to which her markedly slow pace, fine-motor difficulties, and auditory processing deficiencies can impact her measured performance.

Verbal Comprehension

The Verbal Comprehension Index (VCI) attempts to measure verbal concept formation, verbal reasoning, and knowledge acquired from one's environment. Moira's VCI of 98 (45th percentile) is within the Average range, representing adequate ability when compared to same-aged children. Moira performed consistently well on the subtests that are included in this composite score. The first subtest, Similarities, asked her to describe how the meaning of two words was alike. Her performance on this subtest falls in the Average range (Similarities, 37th percentile). The second subtest, Vocabulary, asked her to define words. Her performance on this subtest also falls in the Average range, reflecting adequately developed word knowledge and verbal concept formation (Vocabulary, 50th percentile).

Visual Spatial

The Visual Spatial Index (VSI) attempts to measure the ability to look at visual details and understand visual-spatial relationships in order to construct geometric designs from a model. Moira's VSI of 94 (34th percentile) is within the Average range, representing adequate ability when compared to same-aged children. Moira's scores on the two visual spatial tasks varied. The first subtest, Visual Puzzles, presented her with a completed visual puzzle and asked her to choose three response options to replicate the puzzle. Her performance on this task falls in the Average range (Visual Puzzles, 63rd percentile). The second subtest, Block Design, presented Moira with a constructed model or a picture in the stimulus book and asked her to use red and white blocks to re-create the design within a specified time limit. Her performance on this task falls in the Low Average range (Block Design, 16th percentile). Because she worked slowly her measured performance on this task fails to reflect her actual aptitude. Specifically, Moira arrived at her solution after time limits expired, failing to warrant any credit.

Fluid Reasoning

The Fluid Reasoning Index (FRI) attempts to measure the ability to understand a relationship between visual objects and to solve problems by visually manipulating the information presented. Moira's FRI of 109 (73rd percentile) is within the Average range, representing adequate ability when compared to same-aged children. Moira performed consistently well on the subtests that are included in this composite score. The first subtest, Figure Weights, presented Moira with a visual scale that had missing weights and asked her to select the response option that would balance the scale. Her performance on this subtest is in the Average range (Figure Weights, 63rd percentile). The second subtest, Matrix Reasoning, involves the child looking at an incomplete matrix and selecting the missing portion from five response options. Her performance on this subtest is in the Average range (Matrix Reasoning, 75th percentile). Testing observations of this subtest revealed a second-guessing response style. More specifically, Moira required extended time as she often changed her answer repeatedly before coming to her final answer, suggesting a relative difficulty with anxiety and confidence on this task.

Working Memory Index

The Working Memory Index (WMI) attempts to measure the ability to register, maintain, and manipulate visual and auditory information. Moira's WMI of 88 (21st percentile) is within the Low Average range, representing adequate ability when compared to same-aged children. Moira performed consistently on the subtests that are included in this composite score. The first subtest, Digit Span, is a measure of auditory working memory and has three tasks: to recall numbers that are read aloud in the same order, reverse order, and ascending order. Her performance on this subtest is at the bottom of the Average range (Digit Span, 25th percentile). The second subtest, Picture Span, is a measure of visual working memory and presented Moira with a page of one or more easily identifiable pictures and then asked her to select the pictures that she saw (in order) from a response page. Her performance on this subtest also falls at the bottom of the Average range (Picture Span, 25th percentile). Albeit within normal limits, Moira's WMI index is significantly lower than her other cognitive abilities, suggesting relative difficulties due to her auditory processing deficiencies.

Processing Speed

The Processing Speed Index (PSI) attempts to measure the speed and accuracy of visually identifying information, making decisions, and implementing those decisions. Moira's PSI of 80 (9th percentile) is within the Low Average range, representing a significant weakness when compared to same-aged children. Moira performed consistently on the subtests that are included in this composite score. The first subtest, Coding, involved Moira copying symbols that were paired with simple geometric shapes; using a key, she wrote each symbol in its corresponding box within a specified time limit. Her performance on this subtest falls at the bottom of the Average range (Coding, 25th percentile). The second subtest, Symbol Search, instructed her to scan a search group of symbols and indicate whether a target symbol matched any of the symbols in the search group within a specified time limit. Her performance on this subtest falls in the Borderline range (Symbol Search, 5th percentile). Moira struggled with both subtests; she worked slowly and meticulously, her pencil use was laborious as she complained of hand fatigue. Moira's performances were negatively affected by the time constraints coupled with the fine-motor component.

In sum, current cognitive results reveal Moira is a capable student with good academic potential. Her performance on the WISC-V revealed considerable variability in her cognitive profile. Specifically, she demonstrated adequate problem solving and mental manipulation of visual information. Moira presents with variability between her verbal and nonverbal abilities that is consistent with a DSM-5 diagnosis of Unspecified Neurodevelopmental Disorder (315.9). The pattern of her subtest scores underscores Moira's adequate verbal, visual-spatial, and fluid reasoning skills, while also revealing the extent to which her markedly slow pace, fine-motor difficulties, and auditory processing deficiencies can impact her measured performance.

ACADEMIC ACHIEVEMENT

Wechsler Individual Achievement Test, Third Edition (WIAT-III)

Subtest	*SS*	*Percentile*	*Qualitative*
Mathematics	103	58	Average
Math Problem Solving	102	55	Average
Numerical Operations	104	61	Average
Basic Reading	97	42	Average
Reading Comprehension	105	63	Average
Word Reading	102	55	Average
Pseudoword Decoding	93	32	Average
Essay Composition	123	94	Superior
Grammar & Mechanics	119	90	High Average
Word Count	118	88	High Average
Theme Development & Text Organization	126	96	Superior

Gray Oral Reading Tests, Fifth Edition (GORT-5)

Subtest	*SS*	*Percentile*	*GE*	*Qualitative*
Oral Reading Index	**86**	**18**	—	**Low Average**
Rate	10	50	5.4	Average
Accuracy	7	16	2.7	Low Average
Fluency	8	25	4.0	Average
Comprehension	7	16	3.2	Low Average

Test of Written Language, Third Edition (TOWL-3)

Scale	*SS*	*Percentile*	*Qualitative*
Contextual Conventions	12	75	Average
Contextual Language	9	37	Average
Story Construction	11	63	Average

Woodcock-Johnson Tests of Achievement, Form A, Fourth Edition (WJ-IV)

Subtest	*SS*	*Percentile*	*Qualitative*
Academic Fluency	**96**	**40**	**Average**
Sentence Reading Fluency	92	30	Average
Math Facts Fluency	101	53	Average
Sentence Writing Fluency	97	42	Average

Moira exhibits adequate reading skills, with some variability in the Low Average range secondary to auditory processing deficits. Her basic reading skills are Average (WIAT-III Basic Reading, 42nd percentile). Her foundational reading abilities, including phonetic decoding, are Average (WIAT-III Pseudoword Decoding, 32nd percentile). When asked to read silently, her word reading, including reading rate and accuracy, are within the Average range, reflecting adequately developed sight vocabulary and an ample word bank (WIAT-III Word Reading, 55th percentile; WJ-IV Sentence Reading Fluency, 30th percentile). Moira's reading rate and accuracy were further examined when asked to read aloud. Overall, when reading aloud, Moira's reading rate, accuracy, and reading fluency are negatively affected and measure within the Low Average range (GORT-5 Oral Reading Index, 18th percentile). Moira's ability to answer reading comprehension questions immediately following a short passage falls in the Low Average to Average range (GORT-5 Comprehension, 16th percentile; WIAT-III Reading Comprehension, 63rd percentile). Notably, the stimulus questions had to be repeated more than once for a response. Also, she did mishear questions at the first presentation.

On tests of writing ability, Moira exhibits impressive expressive written language skills. More specifically, Moira's ability to organize her thoughts into a thematically developed presentation ranged from the Average to Very Superior range (TOWL-3 Story Construction, 63rd percentile; WIAT-III Theme Development and Text Organization, 96th percentile). In addition, she performed in the Average range on a task that required her to formulate and write simple sentences about pictures using three given words (WIAT-III Sentence Writing Fluency, 42nd percentile). Finally, Moira demonstrates Average to High Average grammar and mechanics (TOWL-3 Contextual Conventions, 75th percentile; WIAT-III Grammar and Mechanics, 90th percentile).

Moira's mathematical abilities are well developed. She performed in the Average range when asked to exercise her math reasoning skills (WIAT-III Math Problem Solving, 55th percentile), reflecting her intact fluid reasoning and working memory cognitive profile. Her basic mathematical skills are within the Average range (WIAT-III Mathematics, 58th percentile). Similarly, she performed in the Average range on an untimed paper-and-pencil task measuring her ability to perform mathematical computations such as addition, subtraction, multiplication, and division (WIAT-III Numerical Operations, 61st percentile). Her ability to quickly and accurately produce basic mathematical facts falls in the Average range (WJ-IV Math Facts Fluency, 53rd percentile).

In sum, Moira has well-developed academic abilities. She demonstrates academic strengths across reading, writing and math. Specifically on reading tasks, Moira's performance demonstrates her understanding of basic reading fundamentals and higher order reading comprehension skills; her poorer performance reflects, however, auditory processing issues and is not commensurate with her true reading abilities.

AUDITORY PROCESSING

A Test for Auditory Processing Disorder in Adolescents and Adults (SCAN-A)

Subtest	*SS*	*Percentile*	*Qualitative*
Total Test Standard Score	**68**	**2**	**Disordered**
Filtered Words	3	1	Disordered
Auditory-Figure Ground	6	9	Borderline
Competing Words	8	25	Normal
Competing Sentences	3	1	Disordered

Moira's ability to process auditory stimuli was assessed with the SCAN-C. The SCAN-C consists of four subtests, which tap the auditory perceptual skills beyond the peripheral hearing mechanism. The words and sentences are distorted or presented with background noise, which make them difficult for people with auditory processing deficits to hear. Overall, Moira's performance on this task revealed Profoundly Impaired auditory attention and processing abilities with some variability into the Average range (Total Test Standard Score, 2nd percentile).

Moira performed within the Average range when required to decipher words presented simultaneously (Competing Words, 25th percentile). In contrast, she demonstrated difficulty when identifying words that were muffled or presented with background noise (Filtered Words, 1st percentile; Auditory-Figure Ground, 9th percentile). She also demonstrated difficulty when required to decipher sentences presented simultaneously (Competing Sentences, 1st percentile). An error analysis of Moira's performance on these tasks revealed similar sounding words. For example, she identified "bid" for *dad*, "slow" for *low,* and "zuck" for *duck*. Additional errors were due to "no responses," indicating Moira did not sufficiently hear the test items as they were presented.

In sum, Moira's performance on the SCAN-C is consistent to the findings of her auditory and language processing evaluation (Dr. Doe, xx/xx/xx), and further supports the diagnosis of an auditory processing disorder. Moira will have difficulty accurately processing directions with a single exposure. She will also have difficulty accurately processing rapid, unclear speech. Given her auditory processing delays, Moira would benefit from repetition of instructions and instructions clarified, particularly if instructions are given orally, to make sure she understands tasks and requirements before she begins working. She would also benefit from a quiet environment when completing homework and a quiet, separate setting when test taking so as not to become distracted. Moreover, Moira should use an FM unit in the classroom in order to increase clarity and comprehension of auditory input.

LEARNING AND MEMORY

Wide Range Assessment of Memory and Learning, Second Edition (WRAML2)

Subtest	*SS*	*Percentile*	*Qualitative*
Screening Memory	**101**	**53**	**Average**
Verbal Memory	97	42	Average
Story Memory	11	63	Average
Verbal Learning	8	25	Average
Visual Memory	106	66	Average
Design Memory	11	63	Average
Picture Memory	11	63	Average

Rey-Osterreith Complex Figure Test (RCFT), Delayed Recall

Score	SS	Percentile	Qualitative
21/36	96	40	Average

On the WRAML2, Moira's performance on memory and learning tasks is within the Average range (Screening Memory, 53rd percentile). Generally, Moira has a similar ability to recall newly learned verbal information to her ability to recall newly learned visual information.

Moira demonstrated Average verbal memory (Verbal Memory, 42nd percentile). She performed in the Average range on a task in which required her to retell short stories that the examiner read aloud to her (Story Memory, 63rd percentile). Her rote memory ability is Average, as she was able to recall an adequate number of words from a list read aloud to her upon the first trial, and then improved her memory over repeated trials (Verbal Learning, 25th percentile). Similar to verbal memory, Moira's memory for visual information is in the Average range (Visual Memory, 66th percentile). She performed in the Average range when asked to identify missing or changed details in pictures to which she had been exposed to for 10 seconds (Picture Memory, 63rd percentile). She again performed in the Average range when asked to remember and reproduce linear designs (Design Memory, 63rd percentile; RCFT Delayed Recall, 40th percentile).

ATTENTION AND EXECUTIVE FUNCTIONING

Conners Continuous Performance Test, Third Edition (CPT-3)

Measure	T-Score	Guideline
Response Type	55	Balanced
Detectability (d′)	60	Elevated
Error Type	—	—
Omissions	53	Average
Commissions	56	Average
Perseverations	72	Very Elevated
Reaction Time Statistics		
Hit Reaction Time (HRT)	42	A Little Fast
HRT Standard Deviation	58	Average
Variability	58	Average
HRT Block Change	40	Low
HRT Inter-Stimulus Interval (ISI) Change	48	Average

Wisconsin Card Sorting Test (WCST)

		Age-corrected		
WCST scores	*Raw Scores*	*SS*	*T-score*	*Percentiles*
Trials Administered	104	—	—	—
Total Correct	82	—	—	—
Total Errors	22	109	56	73
% Errors	21%	110	57	75
Perseverative Responses	19	97	48	42
% Perseverative Responses	18%	95	47	37
Perseverative Errors	17	97	48	42
% Perseverative Errors	16%	95	47	37
Nonperseverative Errors	5	121	64	92
% Nonperseverative Errors	5%	124	66	95
Conceptual Level Responses	73	—	—	—
% Conceptual Level Responses	70%	105	53	63
Categories Completed	6	—	—	> 16%
Trials to Complete 1st Category	16	—	—	11–16%
Failure to Maintain Set	0	—	—	> 16%
Learning to Learn	1.07	—	—	> 16%

Behavior Assessment System for Children, Third Edition (BASC-3)

Rater	*Mother T-Score*	*Teacher 1 T-Score*	*Teacher 2 T-Score*
Hyperactivity	56	65*	63*
Attention Problems	43	46	49

* At-Risk
** Clinically Significant

Moira was administered the CPT-3 to assess her ability to attend to stimuli. During the 14-minute, 360-trial administration, respondents are required to respond when any letter appears, except the non-target letter "X." Based on Moira's responses on this target decision task, she has a balanced style of responding that is sensitive to both speed and accuracy (Response Type, T-Score = 55). Moira's scores on measures of the CPT-3 indicates she may have issues related to inattentiveness, impulsivity, and sustained attention. Furthermore, Moira's teachers indicate Moira exhibits At-Risk attention problems compared to that of other children her age (BASC-3 TRS Attention Problems, 91st percentile; BASC-3 TRS Attention Problems, 89th percentile). Detectability (d') measures the respondent's ability to differentiate non-targets (i.e., the letter X) from targets (i.e., all other letters). Moira's T-score is 60 and falls in the Elevated range. This result means that her ability to discriminate non-targets from targets was poor when compared to the normative group. Poor ability to differentiate non-targets from targets is an indicator of inattentiveness.

HRT is the mean response speed of correct responses for the whole administration. Moira's T-score is 42 and falls in the A Little Fast range. This result means that her response speed was faster than the normative group's response speed. A faster than normal HRT is often related to impulsivity. Relatedly, Perseverations are random or anticipatory responses. Moira's T-score is 72 and falls in the Very Elevated range. This result means that she made many more perseverative errors when compared to the normative group. Because Moira's response speed (see HRT, above) was A Little Fast, her perseverations are likely caused by impulsivity.

Moira's executive functioning was assessed with the WCST. This task, which involves sorting cards into different categories dependent on feedback regarding errors, assesses the ability to form abstract concepts, to change one's mindset from one category to another, and to learn from one's errors. Her performance on this test indicated that she had difficulty learning from her errors. She completed 6 out of 6 possible categories; however, required significantly more trials to complete a category than would be expected for her age. Overall, her performance reflects cognitive inflexibility and a delay in processing to meet changing task demands.

Moira's performance on attention testing indicates she may have problems with inattentiveness, impulsivity and sustained attention. More specifically, Moira was less able to differentiate targets from non-targets, made more perseverative errors and responded faster. However, according to parent and teacher reports, inattentive symptoms are only significantly noted at school. At this time, Moira does not meet criteria for Attention-Deficit/Hyperactivity Disorder. Teacher observations of Moira's inattentive symptoms are secondary to Moira's auditory processing deficits.

VISUOMOTOR

BEERY Visual-Motor Integration (VMI)

Subtest	*SS*	*Percentile*	*Qualitative*
VMI	86	18	Low Average

Rey-Osterreith Complex Figure Test (RCFT), Copy

Score	*SS*	*Percentile*	*Qualitative*
29/36	101	53	Average

On a measure of her ability to integrate visual and fine motor skills, Moira was able to reproduce a large and detailed figure within the Average range (RCFT Copy, 53rd percentile). As noted previously, her approach to this task was extremely meticulous and effortful. More specifically, she pressed hard onto the paper and stopped to review each mark she made, requiring a significant amount of time to complete the task successfully. In contrast, on a second measure of visual-motor skill integration, Moira's performance is within the Low Average range (VMI, 18th percentile), and represents a more accurate depiction of her fine-motor abilities. This test required her to copy increasingly difficult geometric forms (e.g., lines, circles, and three-dimensional shapes). When compared to the stimulus items, her designs had less-defined and disproportionate angles, as well as missing details in the design. Throughout this task, Moira demonstrated a pressured grip on the pencil, resulting in dark pencil marks and laborious writing. She complained of hand fatigue, and was observed shaking her hand for relief.

PERSONALITY

Behavior Assessment System for Children, Third Edition (BASC-3)

Rater	*Mother PRS-C T-Score*	*Teacher 1 TRS-C T-Score*	*Teacher 2 TRS-C T-Score*
Composites			
Externalizing Problems	48	44	46
Internalizing Problems	59	60*	54
Behavioral Symptoms Index	58	61*	60*
School Problems	—	54	59
Adaptive Skills	35*	41	35*
Scales			
Hyperactivity	43	46	49
Aggression	51	43	46
Conduct Problems	51	43	43
Anxiety	62*	67*	49
Depression	63*	45	45
Somatization	47	60*	64*

Rater	*Mother PRS-C T-Score*	*Teacher 1 TRS-C T-Score*	*Teacher 2 TRS-C T-Score*
Attention Problems	56	65*	63*
Learning Problems	—	43	53
Atypicality	58	93**	82**
Withdrawal	63*	60*	63*
Adaptability	38*	51	51
Social Skills	41	42	28**
Leadership	31*	36*	36*
Study Skills	—	50	41
Functional Communication	36*	30*	29**
Activities of Daily Living	37*	—	—

* At-Risk
** Clinically Significant

In terms of emotional functioning, Moira gives evidence of mild affective disturbance. Although motivated to succeed academically, she is aware of her learning challenges and is experiencing mounting distress and anxiety as a result. Parent reports confirm Moira's considerable anxiety relative to school performance. Her responses to projective testing indicate that she is feeling overwhelmed by internal and external stress, and is more vulnerable than most people to become acutely upset, anxious or even disorganized. In the face of these difficulties, Moira experiences high levels of anxiety and limited self-esteem and self-confidence. Consequently, she shows a tendency toward emotional outbursts including self-deprecating, or avoidance of tasks.

On the Rorschach Inkblot Test, Moira's responses confirmed that she is experiencing some emotional stress that is interfering with her pleasure in life and making her susceptible to becoming anxious. Resolution of issues that are currently troubling her would probably contribute to her feeling better than she does at present. Moreover, Moira demonstrates fairly good abilities to form accurate impressions about herself. Her adequate reality testing constitutes a personality strength; however, as result, Moira is becoming more aware of her academic challenges. Parent and teacher reports reveal Moira is aware when she does not understand the material in class, causing anxiety within the At-Risk range (BASC-3 PRS Anxiety, 89th percentile; BASC-3 TRS Anxiety, 93rd percentile).

In sum, Moira is a sweet, well-mannered, and socially engaging young girl who is experiencing mild affective disturbance. Moira is growing more aware of her learning challenges and is experiencing mounting distress and anxiety as a result. As a consequence, she has little tolerance for uncertainty and ambiguity, feels most comfortable in clearly defined and well-structured situations and favors simple solutions to even complex problems. Despite these difficulties, Moira appears to be highly motivated to perform well. Her strong achievement orientation should serve her in good stead, provided that she receives adequate resources. Her motivation to succeed, coupled with her engaging personality, constitutes a substantial personality strength.

SUMMARY

Moira is an 11-year-old girl referred for an initial neuropsychological evaluation. This consultation is subsequent to recent evaluations in which Moira has been diagnosed with an auditory processing disorder and possible anxiety, depressive, learning, language and attention disorders. Parent and teacher reports indicate that Moira mishears, needs repetition and has trouble following directions. In addition, Moira is distracted by noisy environments, finds it difficult to focus when background noise is present and is disorganized. Moira's intellectual functioning, as assessed by the Wechsler Intelligence Scale for Children—Fifth Edition (WISC-V), is within the Average range (FSIQ = 95, 37th percentile). There was significant score variability between the core cognitive areas that were assessed by the WISC-V; therefore, the FSIQ should be interpreted with caution. Moira presents with variability between her verbal and nonverbal abilities that is consistent with a DSM-5 diagnosis of Unspecified Neurodevelopmental Disorder (315.9). Moira's speed, fine-motor processing and auditory processing deficiencies pose a challenge for her learning and academic performance. She also shows a slowed response rate.

Moira demonstrates academic strengths across reading, writing and math. Specifically on reading tasks, Moira's performance demonstrates her understanding of basic reading fundamentals and higher order reading comprehension skills; her poorer performance reflects, however, auditory processing issues and is not commensurate with her true reading abilities. Despite erratic academic performances due to difficulties with auditory attention and processing, Moira demonstrates impressive fundamental academic skills.

Moira's performance on the auditory processing measures is consistent to the findings of her auditory and language processing evaluation (Dr. Doe, xx/xx/xx), and further supports the diagnosis of an auditory processing disorder. Moira will have difficulty accurately processing directions with a single exposure. She will also have difficulty accurately processing rapid, unclear speech. Given her auditory processing delays, Moira would benefit from repetition of instructions and instructions clarified, particularly if instructions are given orally, to make sure she understands tasks and requirements before she begins working. She would also benefit from a quiet environment when completing homework and a quiet, separate setting when test taking so as not to become distracted. Moreover, Moira should use an FM unit in the classroom in order to increase clarity and comprehension of auditory input.

Moira's performance on attention testing indicates she may have problems with inattentiveness, impulsivity and sustained attention. More specifically, Moira was less able to differentiate targets from non-targets, made more perseverative errors and responded faster. However, according to parent and teacher reports, inattentive symptoms are only significantly noted at school. At this time, Moira does not meet criteria for Attention-Deficit/Hyperactivity Disorder. Teacher observations of Moira's inattentive symptoms are secondary to Moira's auditory processing deficits.

Moira demonstrates fine-motor deficiencies. Fine-motor tasks during the present evaluation were significantly taxing on Moira. More specifically, her approach to pencil-and-paper activities was slow, careful and methodical as she reviewed every mark before advancing to further items. Such tasks required extended time and sustained effort. In addition, she demonstrated a pressured grip on the pencil, resulting in dark pencil marks and laborious writing. Moira complained of hand fatigue, and was observed shaking her hand for relief. Given her fine-motor delays, Moira will benefit from the ability to complete written assignments in a word-processing program.

In terms of emotional functioning, Moira is experiencing mild affective disturbance. She is growing more aware of her learning challenges and is experiencing mounting distress and anxiety as a result. As a consequence, she has little tolerance for uncertainty and ambiguity, feels most comfortable in clearly defined and well-structured situations and favors simple solutions to even complex problems. Despite these difficulties, Moira appears to be highly motivated to perform well. Her strong achievement orientation should serve her in good stead, provided that she receives adequate resources. Her motivation to succeed, coupled with her engaging personality constitutes a substantial personality strength.

DSM-5 DIAGNOSTIC IMPRESSIONS

Moira meets criteria for the following DSM-5 and ICD-10 diagnoses:

315.9; (F89): Unspecified Neurodevelopmental Disorder (NVLD) (Principal Diagnosis)
300.02; (F41.1): Generalized Anxiety Disorder

RECOMMENDATIONS

School Recommendations:

1. It is recommended that Moira attend a small, structured, specialized education program that will address her learning needs. Moira requires a specialized program focused on educating students who have significant language-based learning needs. Moira will require a placement that can also provide her with the individualized support she requires at times in order to guide her attention as well as provide scaffolding to support her academic growth.

   Given her profile and current needs, it will not be appropriate to place Moira in a larger, community school setting. Her needs will not be adequately met in a general education or integrated co-teaching environment. Nor will it be appropriate to place Moira in a self-contained class in a community school, as her specific learning needs will not be met. In such settings, Moira may be placed with inappropriate peer models from a social, behavioral, or learning perspective. These settings do not provide the comprehensive instruction in academic and language skills that Moira requires to make adequate progress. Lastly, it will not be appropriate to place Moira in an academic setting with students who have behavioral or acting out difficulties as this will expose Moira to inappropriate models of behavior as well as exacerbate her anxiety and unduly increase her level of discomfort and emotional distress.
2. Moira is a capable child who has the ability to succeed on a variety of tasks. The following recommendations are offered to assist with Moira's classroom functioning:

   - It is strongly recommended Moira receive 50 percent extended time (i.e., time and a half) on all exams (school and standardized), written assignments, and projects due to her neurocognitive deficits and level of anxiety.
   - It is strongly recommended that Moira complete her exams in a separate location. In the current evaluation Moira performed in the profoundly disordered range on auditory processing measures. Furthermore, she demonstrates distractibility and inattention symptoms in the presence of background noise; a separate setting when test taking will help Moira so as not to become distracted.
   - An FM unit is strongly recommended for use the classroom in order to increase clarity and comprehension of auditory input.

- Moira should be seated where both auditory and visual stimuli are optimally received. Ideally, she should be away from noise and distracting external stimuli.
- It is recommended that Moira be allowed to complete written assignments in a word-processing program. This is due to her fine-motor difficulties.
- The rate of presentation for new material needs to be altered for Moira. She needs additional processing time or time to rehearse the information. Moira needs tasks or information, especially language, broken down into small steps or chunks.
- Individuals like Moira often demonstrate difficulties keeping track of more than one or two steps at a time. Providing a written checklist of steps required to complete a task can serve as an external memory support and alleviate some of the burden on working memory.
- Repetition of instructions or new information is required so that Moira can process and build upon the amount of information captured. Have Moira repeat or paraphrase what she has heard or understood to check for accuracy and comprehension.
- Periodic teacher "check-ins" will be helpful to Moira to ensure comprehension of task demands and encourage goal-focused behavior. Check-ins also can provide opportunities for praise and positive reinforcement.

3. Speech-language therapy is recommended to address her language and auditory deficits.
4. It is recommended that Moira receive an Occupational Therapy evaluation. This is to assess and provide therapy for hand strength, flexibility, and dexterity. During this evaluation, Moira displayed a pressured pencil grip, poor handwriting and self-reported hand fatigue that may have affected performance.

Home Recommendations:

1. It is strongly recommended that Moira consult a psychopharmacologist for a medication stimulant trial to help manage her difficulties with attentiveness, sustained attention, and impulsivity. She will benefit from taking the stimulant prior to executive functioning tasks such as studying or cleaning her room, as well as academic tasks such as reading.
2. It is strongly recommended that Moira participate in psychotherapy treatment to help manage her distress and anxiety. Results of current personality testing reveal she is experiencing some emotional stress that is inter-

fering with her pleasure in life and making her susceptible to becoming anxious or depressed. Resolution of issues that are currently troubling her would contribute to her feeling better than she does at present.

3. It is strongly recommended Moira complete her homework in a quiet location; a separate setting when completing homework will help Moira so as not to become distracted by extraneous auditory stimuli.

______________________________	______________________________
Nechama Sorscher, Ph.D.	Jane Doe
NYS Licensed Psychologist	NYS Certified School Psychologist
License # xxxxxx	Certification # xxxxxxx
Supervisor	Examiner

References

1996 Child and Adolescent Psychiatry Diplomates. (1997). Journal of the American Academy of Child & Adolescent Psychiatry, 36(4), 573. https://doi.org/10.1097/00004583-199704000-00025

Aarnoudse-Moens, C. S. H., Weisglas-Kuperus, N., van Goudoever, J. B., & Oosterlaan, J. (2009). Meta-Analysis of Neurobehavioral Outcomes in Very Preterm and/or Very Low Birth Weight Children. *PEDIATRICS*, *124*(2), 717–728. https://doi.org/10.1542/peds.2008-2816

Acardo, A., Kuder, J., Woodruff, J. (2019) Accommodations and support services preferred by college students with autism spectrum disorder. *Autism*, 20 (3), 574–583.

Adams G. & Carnine, D. (2003) Direct Instruction Handbook of Learning Disabilities, 403–416.

Adams, G. L. & Engleman, S. (1996) Research on direct instruction: 25 years beginning with DISTA Seattle, WA: Ed: Assessment Systems.

Adams, W. & Sheslow, D. (2021) Wide Range Assessment of Memory and Learning–Third Edition, Springer Link, New York.

Allarakhia, H. (2017). Academic Accommodations: They do make a difference. *Journal of Teaching Disability Studies*

Allen, L. B., White, K. S., Barlow, D. H., Shear, M. K., Gorman, J. M., & Woods, S. W. (2009). Cognitive-Behavior Therapy (CBT) for Panic Disorder: Relationship of Anxiety and Depression Comorbidity with Treatment Outcome. *Journal of Psychopathology and Behavioral Assessment*, *32*(2), 185–192. https://doi.org/10.1007/s10862-009-9151-3

Alley, G. R., Deshler, D. D., Clark, F. L., Schumaker, J. B., & Warner, M. M. (1983). Learning Disabilities in Adolescent and Young Adult Populations: Research Implications (Part II). *Focus on Exceptional Children*, *15*(9). https://doi.org/10.17161/foec.v15i9.7456

Alvarado, Camille, and Vania Modesto-Lowe. "Improving Treatment in Minority Children with Attention Deficit/Hyperactivity Disorder." Clinical Pediatrics, vol.

56, no. 2, 20 July 2016, pp. 171–176, 10.1177/0009922816645517. Accessed 10 Oct. 2020.

Alvarez, A. (1992). *Live company: psychoanalytic psychotherapy with autistic, borderline, deprived, and abused children*. Tavistock/Routledge.

American Psychiatric Association. (2013). Diagnostic and Statistical Manual of Mental Disorders. *Diagnostic and Statistical Manual of Mental Disorders*, *5*(5). https://doi.org/10.1176/appi.books.9780890425596

Aminidav, C., & Weller, L. (1995). Effects of country of origin, sex, religiosity and social class on breadth of knowledge of mental retardation. *The British Journal of Development Disabilities*, *41*(80), 48–56. https://doi.org/10.1179/bjdd.1995.007

Anagnostou, E. (2018). Clinical trials in autism spectrum disorder. *Current Opinion in Neurology*, *31*(2), 119–125. https://doi.org/10.1097/wco.0000000000000542

Appelbaum, S. A. (1970). Science and persuasion in the psychological test report. *Journal of Consulting and Clinical Psychology*, *35*(3), 349–355. https://doi.org/10.1037/h0030105

Armstrong, T., & Ebrary, I. (2012). *Neurodiversity in the classroom; strength-based strategies to help students with special needs succeed in school and life*. Ascd.

Armstrong, T. (2010). *Neurodiversity; discovering the extraordinary gifts of autism, ADHD, dyslexia, and other brain differences*. Da Capo Lifelong.

Aron, L. (1991). The patient's experience of the analyst's subjectivity. *Psychoanalytic Dialogues*, *1*(1), 29–51. https://doi.org/10.1080/10481889109538884

Aron, L. (1996). *A meeting of minds: Mutuality in psychoanalysis.* Analytic Press, Inc.

Artiles, A. (Host). (2021, May 24). How disability intersects with race [Audio podcast episode] in *School's In.* Stanford University Graduate School of Education. https://ed.stanford.edu/news/how-disability-intersects-race-language-and-social-class

Anthes, E. (2023, March 23). *Autism prevalence rises again, study finds*. The New York Times. https://www.nytimes.com/2023/03/23/health/autism-children-diagnosis.html

Autism Speaks. "Autism Speaks." Autism Speaks, 2018, www.autismspeaks.org/.

Backman, A., Mellblom, A., Norman-Claesson, E., Keith-Bodros, G., Frostvittra, M., Bölte, S., & Hirvikoski, T. (2018). Internet-delivered psychoeducation for older adolescents and young adults with autism spectrum disorder (SCOPE): An open feasibility study. *Research in Autism Spectrum Disorders*, *54*, 51–64. https://doi.org/10.1016/j.rasd.2018.07.001

Baker, D., & Scanlon, D. (2016). Student Perspectives on academic accommodations. *Exceptionality*, *24*(2), 93–108. https://doi.org/10.1080/09362835.2015.1064411

Ballentine, K. (2019). Understanding racial differences in diagnosing ODD versus ADHD using Critical race Theory. *Families in society-The Journal of Contemporary Social Services*, *100*(3), 282–292. https://doi.org/10.1177/1044389419842765

Barendse, M. E., Flannery, J., Cavanagh, C., Aristizabal, M., Becker, S. P., Berger, E., Breaux, R., Campione-Barr, N., Church, J. A., Crone, E. A., Dahl, R. E., Dennis-Tiwary, T. A., Dvorsky, M. R., Dziura, S. L., Van De Groep, S., Ho, T. C., Killoren, S. E., Langberg, J. M., Larguinho, T. L., . . . Pfeifer, J. H. (2022). Longitudinal Change in Adolescent Depression and Anxiety Symptoms from before to during the COVID-19 Pandemic. *Journal of Research on Adolescence*, *33*(1), 74–91. https://doi.org/10.1111/jora.12781

Barkley, R. A. (2018). *Attention-deficit hyperactivity disorder: A handbook for diagnosis and treatment*. The Guilford Press.

Barzegary, L., & Zamini, S. (2011). The Effect of Play Therapy on Children with ADHD. *Procedia–Social and Behavioral Sciences*, *30*, 2216–2218. https://doi.org/10.1016/j.sbspro.2011.10.432

Bearss, K., Johnson, C., Smith, T., Lecavalier, L., Swiezy, N., Aman, M., McAdam, D. B., Butter, E., Stillitano, C., Minshawi, N., Sukhodolsky, D. G., Mruzek, D. W., Turner, K., Neal, T., Hallett, V., Mulick, J. A., Green, B., Handen, B., Deng, Y., & Dziura, J. (2015). Effect of Parent Training vs Parent Education on Behavioral Problems in Children with Autism Spectrum Disorder. *JAMA*, *313*(15), 1524. https://doi.org/10.1001/jama.2015.3150

Becerra, T. A., Von Ehrenstein, O. S., Heck, J. E., Olsen, J., Arah, O. A., Jeste, S., Rodriguez, M., & Ritz, B. (2014). Autism Spectrum Disorders and Race, Ethnicity, and Nativity: A Population-Based Study. *Pediatrics*, *134*(1), e63–e71. https://doi.org/10.1542/peds.2013-3928

Beebe, D. W., & Risi, S. (2003). Treatment of adolescents and young adults with high-functioning autism or Asperger syndrome. In M. A. Reinecke, F. M. Dattilio, & A. Freeman (Eds.), *Cognitive therapy with children and adolescents: A casebook for clinical practice* (pp. 369–401). The Guilford Press.

Beery, K. E. (1997). The Beery-Buktenica Developmental Test of Visual-Motor Integration: Administration, Scoring and Teaching Manual (4th Ed). Parsippany, NJ: Modern Curriculum Press.

Bender, L. (1946) B*ender Motor Gestalt Test and Manual of Instructions*. American Orthopsychiatric Association, APA

Bender, W. N., & Wall, M. E. (1994). Social-Emotional Development of Students with Learning Disabilities. *Learning Disability Quarterly*, *17*(4), 323–341. https://doi.org/10.2307/1511128

Bennett-levy, J., Klein-bonschate, M. A., Batchelor, J., McCarter, R., Walton, N. (1994) Encounters with Anna Thompson: The consumer's experience of neuropsychological assessment. *Clinical Neuropsychologist*, 8:2, 219–238.

Bhattacharjee, Dipanjan & Rai, Altul & Singh, Narendra & Kumar, Pradeep & Munda, Sanjay & Das, Basudeb. (2011). Psychoeducation: A Measure to Strengthen Psychiatric Treatment. *Industrial psychiatry journal. 14*. 33–39.

Bigelow, B. J. (2006). There's an elephant in the room: The impact of early poverty and neglect on intelligence and common learning disorders in children, adolescents, and their parents. *Developmental Disabilities Bulletin*, *34*(1 & 2), 177–215.

Bioulac, S., Arfi, L., & Bouvard, M. (2008). Attention deficit/hyperactivity disorder and video games: A comparative study of hyperactive and control children. *European Psychiatry*, *23*(2), 134–141. https://doi.org/10.1016/j.eurpsy.2007.11.002

Bitsko, Rebecca H., et al. "Mental Health Surveillance among Children—United States, 2013–2019." *MMWR Supplements*, vol. 71, no. 2, 25 Feb. 2022, pp. 1–42, 10.15585/mmwr.su7102a1.

Brandenburg, J. E., Holman, L. K., Apkon, S. D., Houtrow, A. J., Rinaldi, R., & Sholas, M. G. (2020). School reopening during COVID-19 pandemic: Considering students with disabilities. *Journal of Pediatric Rehabilitation Medicine*, *13*(3), 425–431. https://doi.org/10.3233/prm-200789

Braswell, L., & Bloomquist, M. L. (1991). *Cognitive-behavioral therapy with ADHD children: child, family, and school interventions*. Guilford Press.

Brendli, K.RScott, L. A., Xu, Y., Thoma, C., Holzberg, D. (2021). Effects of a self-advocacy intervention on abilities of black college students with intellectual and developmental disabilities to request academic accommodations. *Inclusion*, 9 (3), 225–240.

Brock, A., & Shute, R. (2001). Group coping skills program for parents of children with dyslexia and other learning disabilities. *Australian Journal of Learning Disabilities*, *6*(4), 15–25. https://doi.org/10.1080/19404150109546683

Broucek, F. J. (1991). *Shame and the self.* Guilford Press.

Bryan, T. (1991). Social Problems in Learning Disabilities in *Learning about Learning Disabilities*. B. Wong Ed. Academic Press, CA.

Bryant, B (2012) *Gray Oral Reading Tests–Fifth Edition* (GORT-5) Austin, TX: Pro-Ed.

Buchen, N., Langberg, J. M., & Becker, S. P. (2021). Prospective impact of Covid-19 on mental health functioning in adolescents with and without ADHD: Protective role of emotion regulation abilities. *Journal of Child Psychology and Psychiatry*, *62*(9), 1132–1139. https://doi.org/10.1111/jcpp.13382

Buchholz, E. S. (1987). The legacy from childhood: Considerations for treatment of the adult with learning disabilities. *Psychoanalytic Inquiry*, *7*(3), 431–452.

Buechler, S. (2008). *Making a difference in patients' lives: Emotional experience in the therapeutic setting.* Routledge.

Bush, G. (2011). Cingulate, frontal, and parietal cortical dysfunction in attention-deficit/hyperactivity disorder. *Biological Psychiatry*, *69*(12), 1160–1167. https://doi.org/10.1016/j.biopsych.2011.01.022

Byrnes, M. A. (2008) Educators' interpretations of ambiguous accommodations. *Remedial and Special Education.* 29 (5) 306–315,

Calarco, J. M. (2018). *Negotiating Opportunities.* New York: Oxford University Press.

Capozzi, F., Casini, M. P., Romani, M., De Genaro, L., Giampaolo, N,, Solano, L. (2008) Psychiatric Comorbidity in Learning Disorder: An analysis of Family Variables. *Child Psychiatry Human Development.* 39:101–110.

Carney, J. K. (2002). Self- and interactive regulation: Treating a patient with AD/HD. *Psychoanalytic Inquiry*, *22*(3), 355–371. https://doi.org/10.1080/07351692209348992

Carney, R. N., & Levin, J. R. (2002). Pictorial illustrations still improve students' learning from text. *Educational psychology review*, *14*(1), 5–26.

Carpenter-Song, E. (2008). Caught in the psychiatric net: Meanings and experiences of ADHD, pediatric bipolar disorder and mental health treatment among a diverse group of families in the United States. *Culture, Medicine, and Psychiatry*, *33*(1), 61–85. https://doi.org/10.1007/s11013-008-9120-4

Carr, T. (2013). Autism diagnostic observation schedule. In *Springer eBooks* (pp. 349–356). https://doi.org/10.1007/978-1-4419-1698-3_896

Castellanos, F. X., Giedd, J. N., Marsh, W., Hamburger, S., Vaituzis, A. C., Dickstein, D. P., Sarfatti, S. E., Vauss, Y. C., Snell, J., Lange, N., Kaysen, D., Krain, A. L., Ritchie, G. F., Rajapakse, J. C., & Rapoport, J. L. (1996). Quantitative Brain magnetic resonance Imaging in Attention-Deficit Hyperactivity Disorder. *Archives of General Psychiatry*, *53*(7), 607. https://doi.org/10.1001/archpsyc.1996.01830070053009

Centers for Disease Control and Prevention. (2018). Data and statistics about ADHD. Centers for Disease Control and Prevention. https://www.cdc.gov/ncbddd/adhd/data.html

Champeaux, H., Mangiavacchi, L., Marchetta, F., & Piccoli, L. (2022). Child development and distance learning in the age of COVID-19. *Review of Economics of the Household, 20*(3), 659–685. https://doi.org/10.1007/s11150-022-09606-w

Chawla, N., Tom, A., Sen, M. S., & Sagar, R. (2021). Psychological Impact of COVID-19 on Children and Adolescents: A Systematic Review. *Indian journal of psychological medicine*, *43*(4), 294–299. https://doi.org/10.1177/02537176211021789

Chused, A. (1991). The transference neurosis in child analysis. *Saying goodbye: A casebook of termination in child and adolescent analysis and therapy*, 233–265.

Clone et al., (2011) Psychodynamic play therapy with a six-year-old African American boy

Cohen, J. (1986). Learning Disabilities and Psychological Development in Childhood and Adolescence. *Churchill Forum* Vol. 8 No. 4

Cohen, M. J., Morgan, A. M., Vaughn, M. (1999). Verbal fluency in children: Developmental issues and differential validity in distinguishing children with attention-deficit hyperactivity disorders and two subtypes of dyslexia. *Archives Clinical Neuropsychology*. 14:433–443.

Cohen, N.J, Davine, M. Horodezky, N., (1993) Unsuspected language impairment in psychiatrically disturbed children: Prevalence and language and behavioral characteristics. *Journal of the American Academy of Child and Adolescent Psychiatry.* 32:595–603.

Coker, T. R., Elliott, M. N., Toomey, S. L., Schwebel, D. C., Cuccaro, P., Emery, S. T., Davies, S. L., Visser, S. N., & Schuster, M. A. (2016). Racial and ethnic disparities in ADHD diagnosis and treatment. *Pediatrics*, *138*(3), e20160407. https://doi.org/10.1542/peds.2016-0407

Colvin, M. K., Forchelli, G. A., Reese, K. L., Capawana, M. R., Beery, C. S., Murphy, J., Doyle, A. E., O'Keefe, S. M., & Braaten, E. B. (2022). Neuropsychology consultation to identify learning disorders in children and adolescents: a proposal based on lessons learned during the COVID-19 pandemic. *Child neuropsychology; a journal on normal and abnormal development in childhood and adolescence*, *28*(5), 671–688. https://doi.org/10.1080/09297049.2021.2005010

Connie E. Morrow, Jan L. Culbertson, Veronica H. Accornero, Lihua Xue, James C. Anthony & Emmalee S. Bandstra (2006) Learning Disabilities and Intellectual Functioning in School-Aged Children With Prenatal Cocaine Exposure, Developmental Neuropsychology, 30:3, 905-931, DOI: 10.1207/s15326942dn3003_8

Connors, C. K. (1995). *Connors' Continuous Performance Test.* North Tonawanda, NY: Multi Health Systems.

Constantino, J. N. & Gruber, C. P. (2012) *Social Responsiveness Scale.* Second Edition. (SRS-2). Torrance, CA: Western Psychological Services.

Conway, F. (2017). *Cultivating Compassion: A psychodynamic understanding of attention deficit hyperactivity disorder.* Lanham, MD: Rowman & Littlefield.

Conway, F., & Gensler, D. (2014). Trouble Paying Attention. In *Attention deficit hyperactivity disorder integration of cognitive, neuropsychological, and psychodynamic perspectives in Psychotherapy*. London: Routledge.

Coutinho, M. J., Oswald, D. P., & Best, A. M. (2002). The influence of sociodemographics and gender on the disproportionate identification of minority students as having learning disabilities. *Remedial and Special Education*, *23*(1), 49–59. https://doi.org/10.1177/074193250202300107

Cowan, N. (2008). Chapter 20. What are the differences between long-term, short-term, and working memory? In *Progress in Brain Research* (pp. 323–338). https://doi.org/10.1016/s0079-6123(07)00020-9

Dagnan, D., Jackson, I., & Eastlake, L. (2018). A systematic review of cognitive behavioural therapy for anxiety in adults with intellectual disabilities. *Journal of Intellectual Disability Research*, *62*(11), 974–991. https://doi.org/10.1111/jir.12548

Dagnan, D., Jahoda, A. & Kroese, B. S. (2016) *Cognitive Behavior Therapy in The Handbook of Intellectual Disability and Clinical Psychology Practice*, Routledge

Damiano, C. R., Mazefsky, C. A., White, S. W., & Dichter, G. S. (2014). Future directions for research in autism spectrum disorders. *Journal of clinical child and adolescent psychology; the official journal for the Society of Clinical Child and Adolescent Psychology, American Psychological Association, Division 53*, *43*(5), 828–843. https://doi.org/10.1080/15374416.2014.945214

Daneman, M., & Carpenter, P. A. (1980). Individual differences in working memory and reading. *Journal of Verbal Learning & Verbal Behavior, 19*(4), 450–466. https://doi.org/10.1016/S0022-5371(80)90312-6

Danial, J. T., & Wood, J. J. (2013). Cognitive Behavioral Therapy for Children With Autism. *Journal of Developmental & Behavioral Pediatrics*, *34*(9), 702–715. https://doi.org/10.1097/dbp.0b013e31829f676c

Danielson, M. L., Bitsko, R. H., Ghandour, R. M., Holbrook, J., Kogan, M. D., & Blumberg, S. J. (2018). Prevalence of Parent-Reported ADHD Diagnosis and Associated Treatment among U.S. children and Adolescents, 2016. *Journal of Clinical Child and Adolescent Psychology*, *47*(2), 199–212. https://doi.org/10.1080/15374416.2017.1417860

Datlen, G. W., & Pandolfi, C. (2020). Developing an online art therapy group for Learning Disabled Young Adults using WhatsApp. *International Journal of Art Therapy*, *25*(4), 192–201. https://doi.org/10.1080/17454832.2020.1845758

Davenport, M., Mazurek, M. O., Brown, A. M., & McCollom, E. M. (2018). A systematic review of cultural considerations and adaptation of social skills interventions for individuals with autism spectrum disorder. *Research in Autism Spectrum Disorders*, *52*, 23–33. https://doi.org/10.1016/j.rasd.2018.05.003

David, H. (2017). A double label: Learning disabilities and emotional problems among gifted children. *International Letters of Social and Humanistic Sciences,* 75, 22–31.

Davidson, C. J., Lodge, K., & Kam, A. (2021). The impact of the COVID-19 pandemic on Autistic Adults—A survey. *Advances in Autism, 7*(4), 311–321. https://doi.org/10.1108/aia-10-2020-0057

De Bellis, M. D., & Zisk, A. (2014). The biological effects of childhood trauma. *Child and Adolescent Psychiatric Clinics of North America, 23*(2), 185–222. https://doi.org/10.1016/j.chc.2014.01.002

De Figueiredo, C. S., Sandre, P. C., Portugal, L. C., Mázala-de-Oliveira, T., da Silva Chagas, L., Raony, Í., Ferreira, E. S., Giestal-de-Araujo, E., dos Santos, A. A., & Bomfim, P. O.-S. (2021). Covid-19 pandemic impact on children and adolescents' mental health: Biological, environmental, and social factors. *Progress in Neuro-Psychopharmacology and Biological Psychiatry, 106*, 110171. https://doi.org/10.1016/j.pnpbp.2020.110171

Decker, T. W., Polloway, E. A., & Decker, B. B. (1985). Help for the LD college student. *Academic Therapy,* 20 (3), 339–345.

Dekker, M. C. & Koot, H.M (2003). DSM-IV disorders in children with borderline to moderate intellectual disability: Prevalence and impacts. *Journal of American Academy of Child and Adolescent Psychiatry* 42:915–22

Delis, D. C., Kaplan, E. & Kramer, J. H. (2001) *Delis-Kaplan Executive Function System (D-KEFS).* PsycTESTS

Deshler, D. D. (2005). Adolescents with Learning Disabilities: Unique Challenges and Reasons for Hope. *Learning Disability Quarterly, 28*(2), 122–124. https://doi.org/10.2307/1593609

Dietmut Niedecken. (2003). *Nameless; understanding learning disability.* Brunner-Routledge.

Donders J. (2020). The incremental value of neuropsychological assessment: A critical review. *The Clinical neuropsychologist, 34*(1), 56–87. https://doi.org/10.1080/13854046.2019.1575471

Donofrio, N., Piatt, A., Whelihan, W., & DiCarlo, M. (1999). Neuropsychological test feedback: Consumer evaluation and perceptions. *Archives of Clinical Neuropsychology, 14*(8), 721.

Donohue, M. R., Childs, A. W., Richards, M., & Robins, D. L. (2017). Race influences parent report of concerns about symptoms of autism spectrum disorder. *Autism, 23*(1), 100–111. https://doi.org/10.1177/1362361317722030

dosReis, S., Butz, A., Lipkin, P. H., Anixt, J. S., Weiner, C. L., & Chernoff, R. (2006). Attitudes about stimulant medication for attention-deficit/hyperactivity disorder among African American families in an inner-city community. *The Journal of Behavioral Health Services & Research, 33*(4), 423–430. https://doi.org/10.1007/s11414-006-9038-y

Douglas, V. I. (1972) Stop, Look and Listen: The problem of sustained attention and impulse control in hyperactive and normal children. *Canadian Journal Of Behavioral Science.*4:259-81.

DuPaul, G. J. (2007). School-based interventions for students with attention deficit hyperactivity disorder: Current status and Future Directions. *School Psychology Review, 36*(2), 183–194. https://doi.org/10.1080/02796015.2007.12087939

DuPaul, G. J., Weyandt, L. L., O'Dell, S. M., & Varejao, M. (2009). College students with ADHD. *Journal of Attention Disorders*, *13*(3), 234–250. https://doi.org/10.1177/1087054709340650

Durkin, M. S., Maenner, M. J., Meaney, F. J., Levy, S. E., DiGuiseppi, C., Nicholas, J. S., Kirby, R. S., Pinto-Martin, J., & Schieve, L. A. (2010). Socioeconomic Inequality in the Prevalence of Autism Spectrum Disorder: Evidence from a U.S. Cross-Sectional Study. *PLOS ONE*, *5*(7), e11551. https://doi.org/10.1371/journal.pone.0011551

Dyches, T. T., Wilder, L. K., Sudweeks, R. R., Obiakor, F. E., & Algozzine, B. (2004). Multicultural issues in autism. *Journal of Autism and Developmental Disorders*, *34*(2), 211–222. https://doi.org/10.1023/b:jadd.0000022611.80478.73

Dyson, L. (2010). Unanticipated Effects of Children with Learning Disabilities on Their Families. *Learning Disability Quarterly*, *33*(1), 43–55. https://doi.org/10.1177/073194871003300104

Ehrenberg, D. B. (1992). *The intimate edge: Extending the reach of psychoanalytic interaction.* W.W. Norton & Co.

Emerson, E., Azmi, S., Hatton, C., Caine, A., Parrott, R., & Wolstenholme, J. (1997). Is there an increased prevalence of severe learning disabilities among british asians? *Ethnicity & Health*, *2*(4), 317–321. https://doi.org/10.1080/13557858.1997.9961840

Epp, K. M. (2008). Outcome-based evaluation of a social skills program using art therapy and group therapy for children on the autism spectrum. *Children & Schools*, *30*(1), 27–36. https://doi.org/10.1093/cs/30.1.27

Ethnicity and equality. (2021, November 17). Foundation for People With Learning Disabilities. https://www.learningdisabilities.org.uk/learning-disabilities/our-work/rights-equality/ethnicity-and-equality

Exner, J. E. (1993) *The Rorschach: A Comprehensive System: Basic Foundations. Volume 1* John Wiley & Sons.

Fairman, K. A., Peckham, A. M., & Sclar, D. A. (2017). Diagnosis and treatment of ADHD in the United States: Update by gender and race. *Journal of Attention Disorders*, *24*(1), 10–19. https://doi.org/10.1177/1087054716688534

Fajardo, B. (1988). Constitution in infancy: Implications for early development and psychoanalysis. *Progress in Self Psychology*, *4*, 91–100.

Farooq, S., & Fear, C. (2003). Working through interpreters. *Advances in Psychiatric Treatment*, *9*(2), 104–109. https://doi.org/10.1192/apt.9.2.104

Farzi Vanestanagh, F., Taklavi, S., & Gaffari, A. (2020). The Effectiveness of Self-Compassion Education on the Shame and Guilt of Mothers of Children with Learning Disorders. *Journal of Health*, *11*(3), 422–431. https://doi.org/10.29252/j.health.11.3.422

Fatimilehin, I., & Nadirshaw, Z. (2010). A cross-cultural study of parental attitudes and beliefs about Learning Disability (Mental Handicap). *Mental Handicap Research*, *7*(3), 202–227. https://doi.org/10.1111/j.1468-3148.1994.tb00127.x

Fegert, J. M., Vitiello, B., Plener, P. L., & Clemens, V. (2020). Challenges and burden of the Coronavirus 2019 (COVID-19) pandemic for child and adolescent mental health: a narrative review to highlight clinical and research needs in the acute phase and the long return to normality. *Child and adolescent psychiatry and mental health*, *14*, 20. https://doi.org/10.1186/s13034-020-00329-3

Ferenczi, Sándor (1988) Confusion of Tongues between Adults and the Child, Contemporary Psychoanalysis, 24:2, 196 206, DOI: 10.1080/00107530.1988.10746234

Fernando, S. (2016). *Race and culture in psychiatry*. London: Routledge.

Ferrell, D. & Marshak, L. (2004). *Up close and personal: University students with disabilities, transition planning and career choices*. Paper presented at the Fifth International Conference on Higher Education and Disability in Innsbruck, Austria.

Ferrin, M., Moreno-Granados, J. M., Salcedo-Marin, M. D., Ruiz-Veguilla, M., Perez-Ayala, V., & Taylor, E. (2013). Evaluation of a psychoeducation programme for parents of children and adolescents with ADHD: immediate and long-term effects using a blind randomized controlled trial. *European Child & Adolescent Psychiatry*, *23*(8), 637–647. https://doi.org/10.1007/s00787-013-0494-7

Ferrin, M., Perez-Ayala, V., El-Abd, S., Lax-Pericall, T., Jacobs, B., Bilbow, A., & Taylor, E. (2016). A Randomized Controlled Trial Evaluating the Efficacy of a Psychoeducation Program for Families of Children and Adolescents With ADHD in the United Kingdom: Results After a 6-Month Follow-Up. *Journal of Attention Disorders*, *24*(5), 768–779. https://doi.org/10.1177/1087054715626509

Finn, S. E., & Tonsager, M. E. (1997). Information-gathering and therapeutic models of assessment: Complementary paradigms. *Psychological assessment*, *9*(4), 374.

Fitzgerald, G. E. (1994). Using the computer with students with emotional and behavioral disorders. *Technology and Disability*, *3*(2), 87–99. https://doi.org/10.3233/tad-1994-3204

Flavell, J. H. (1979). Metacognition and cognitive monitoring: A new area of cognitive developmental inquiry. *American Psychologist.* 34 (10) 906–911.

Florell, D. & Strait, A. (2020) *Academic Accommodations and Modifications in The Clinical Guide to Assessment and Treatment of Childhood Learning and Attention Problems.* M. Martel Ed Academic Press, San Diego, CA.

Flynn, S., Caton, S., Gillooly, A., Bradshaw, J., Hastings, R. P., Hatton, C., Jahoda, A., Mulhall, P., Todd, S., Beyer, S., & Taggart, L. (2021). The experiences of adults with learning disabilities in the UK during the COVID-19 pandemic: Qualitative results from Wave 1 of the coronavirus and people with learning disabilities study. *Tizard Learning Disability Review*, *26*(4), 224–229. https://doi.org/10.1108/tldr-09-2021-0027

Fogler, J. M., Weaver, A. L., Katusic, S., Voigt, R. G., Barbares, W. J., (2020). Recalled experiences of bullying and victimization in a longitudinal, population-based birth cohort: The influence of ADHD and Co-occurring psychiatric disorder. *Journal of Attention Disorders* 10:1177.

Ford, T., John, A., & Gunnell, D. (2021). Mental health of children and young people during pandemic. *BMJ (Clinical research ed.)*, *372*, n614. https://doi.org/10.1136/bmj.n614

Forlin, C. (2012). *Future directions for inclusive teacher education: An international perspective*. London: Routledge.

Fovet, F. (2007). Using distance learning electronic tools within the class to engage ADHD students: A key to inclusion?. Proceedings–Frontiers in Education Conference, FIE. F3D-15. 10.1109/FIE.2007.4417842.

Fox, C. L., & Forbing, S. E. (1991). Overlapping symptoms of substance abuse and learning handicaps: Implications for educators. *Journal of Learning Disabilities*, *24*(1), 24–31. https://doi.org/10.1177/002221949102400106

Franceschini, S., Gori, S., Ruffino, M., Viola, S., Molteni, M., & Facoetti, A. (2013). Action video games make dyslexic children read better. *Current Biology*, *23*(6), 462–466. https://doi.org/10.1016/j.cub.2013.01.044

Fried, P. A., Watkinson, B., & Siegel, L. S. (1997). Reading and language in 9- to 12-year olds prenatally exposed to cigarettes and marijuana. *Neurotoxicology and Teratology*, *19*(3), 171–183. https://doi.org/10.1016/s0892-0362(97)00015-9

Furfaro, H. (2017, November 20). Race, class contribute to disparities in autism diagnoses. *Spectrum | Autism Research News*. https://www.spectrumnews.org/news/race-class-contribute-disparities-autism-diagnoses/

Galaburda, A. M., Sherman, G. F., Rosen, G. D., Aboitiz, F., & Geschwind, N. (1985). Developmental dyslexia: Four consecutive patients with cortical anomalies. *Annals of Neurology*, *18*(2), 222–233. https://doi.org/10.1002/ana.410180210

Galea, S., Merchant, R. M., & Lurie, N. (2020). The mental health consequences of COVID-19 and physical distancing. *JAMA Internal Medicine*, *180*(6), 817. https://doi.org/10.1001/jamainternmed.2020.1562

Gantman, A., Karp, S. K., Oreski, K., & Langeson, E. D. (2012). Social skills training for young adults with high functioning Autism Spectrum Disorder: A randomized control pilot study. *Journal of Autism and Developmental Disorders* 42(6) 1094–1103.

Gardner, M. F. (2000) *Expressive One-Word Picture Vocabulary-2000* Edition. Novato, CA: Academic Therapy Publications.

Gardner, R. A. (1980). What Every Psychoanalyst Should Know about Minimal Brain Dysfunction. *Journal of the American Academy of Psychoanalysis.* 8(3).

Geffner, D. S., & Ross-Swain, D. (2019). *Auditory processing disorders: Assessment, management, and treatment.* Plural Publishing, Inc.

Gensler, D. (1993). Learning Disability in Adulthood. *Contemporary Psychoanalysis*, *29*(4), 673–692. https://doi.org/10.1080/00107530.1993.10746831

Gensler, D. (2011). Trouble paying attention. *Journal of Infant, Child & Adolescent Psychotherapy, 10*(1), 103–115. https://doi.org/10.1080/15289168.2011.575713

Gerber, P. J. (2011). The impact of learning disabilities on adulthood. A review of the evidence-based literature for research and practices in adult education. *Journal of Learning Disabilities.* 45 (1) 31–46.

Germano, E., Gagliano, A., Curatolo, P. (2010) Comorbidity of ADHD and Dyslexia. *Developmental Neuropsychology* 35 (5): 475–93.

Gersten, R., Woodward, J., & Darch, C. (1986). Direct Instruction: A Research-Based Approach to Curriculum design and teaching. *Exceptional Children*, *53*(1), 17–31. https://doi.org/10.1177/001440298605300102

Gilmore, K. (2000). A psychoanalytic perspective on attention-deficit/hyperactivity disorder. *Journal of the American Psychoanalytic Association*, *48*(4), 1259–1293. https://doi.org/10.1177/00030651000480040901

Gizer, I. R., Ficks, C., & Waldman, I. D. (2009). Candidate gene studies of ADHD: A Meta-Analytic Review. *Human Genetics*, *126*(1), 51–90. https://doi.org/10.1007/s00439-009-0694-x

Goldfus, C (2012). Intervention through neurocognitive development: A case study of a student with dyslexia and combined Attention Deficit Disorder (ADD). *Journal of Language and Culture* 3 (3) 55–66.

Goldstein, G. & Golden, H. (2011). Sabert Basescu: Selected papers on human nature and psychoanalysis. Sabert Basescu: Selected Papers on Human Nature and Psychoanalysis. 1–203. 10.4324/9780203868669.

Golstein, G., Minshaw, N. J. & Siegel, D. J. (1994) Age Differences in Academic Achievement high-functioning autistic individuals. Journal of Clinical and Experimental Neuropsychology, 16, 671–680.

Gordon, K., Murin, M., Baykaner, O., Roughan, L., Livermore-Hardy, V., Skuse, D., & Mandy, W. (2014). A randomised controlled trial of PEGASUS, a psychoeducational programme for young people with high-functioning autism spectrum disorder. *Journal of Child Psychology and Psychiatry*, *56*(4), 468–476. https://doi.org/10.1111/jcpp.12304

Gorske, T. T. (2008). Therapeutic neuropsychological assessment: A humanistic model and case example. *Journal of Humanistic Psychology*, *48*(3), 320–339.

Gotham, K., Risi, S., Pickles, A., Lord, C. (2006). The Autism Diagnostic Observation Schedule Journal of Autism and Developmental Disorders.

Grabovschi, C., Loignon, C., & Fortin, M. (2013). Mapping the concept of vulnerability related to health care disparities: a scoping review. *BMC Health Services Research*, *13*(1). https://doi.org/10.1186/1472-6963-13-94

Green, C. S., & Bavelier, D. (2003). Action video game modifies visual selective attention. *Nature*, *423*(6939), 534–537. https://doi.org/10.1038/nature01647

Greenberg, T. M. (2016) Gray Areas: When Illness may be particularly impacted by psychological variables in Psychodynamic Perspectives on aging and illness. Springer, Cham.

Grolnick, W. & Ryan, R. (1990). Self-perceptions, motivation and achievement of children with learning disabilities:a multiple group comparison study. *Journal of Learning Disabilities*. 23:177–184.

Guo, L., Danielson, M., Cogan, L., Hines, L., & Armour, B. (2018). Treatment patterns and costs among children aged 2 to 17 years with ADHD in New York State Medicaid in 2013. *Journal of Attention Disorders*, *25*(4), 463–472. https://doi.org/10.1177/1087054718816176

Hadley, W. M. (2007). The necessity of academic accommodations for first year college students with learning disabilities. *Journal of College Admissions*. 195, 9–13.

Hallowell, Edward M, and John J Ratey. *Driven to Distraction; Recognizing and Coping with Attention Deficit Disorder from Childhood through Adulthood*. New York, Simon & Schuster, 1995.

Halpern-Manners, A., McLeod, J. D., Anderson, E. M., & Ekl, E. A. (2022). Covid-19 and changes in college student educational expectations and health by disability status. *SSM–Population Health*, *19*, 101195. https://doi.org/10.1016/j.ssmph.2022.101195

Hamilton, A. M., Fowler, J. L., Hersh, B., Austin, C. A., Finn, S. E., Tharinger, D. J., & Arora, P. (2009). "Why won't my parents help me?": Therapeutic Assessment of a child and her family. *Journal of Personality Assessment*, *91*(2), 108–120.

Hammill, D. D. & Larsen, S. C. (1996). *Test of Written Language* (3rd Ed) Los Angeles, CA Western Psychological Services

Hardre, P. L., & Reeve, J. (2003). A motivational model of rural students' intentions to persist in, versus drop out of, high school. *Journal of Educational Psychology*, *95*(2), 347–356. https://doi.org/10.1037/0022-0663.95.2.347

Harper, K. (2017, January 12). *5 things to know about racial and ethnic disparities in special education–Child Trends*. ChildTrends. https://www.childtrends.org/publications/5-things-to-know-about-racial-and-ethnic-disparities-in-special-education

Harpin, V., Mazzone, L., Raynaud, J., Kahle, J., & Hodgkins, P. (2013). Long-Term outcomes of ADHD. *Journal of Attention Disorders*, *20*(4), 295–305. https://doi.org/10.1177/1087054713486516

Harrison, A. J., Long, K. A., Tommet, D., & Jones, R. N. (2017). Examining the role of race, ethnicity, and gender on social and behavioral ratings within the autism Diagnostic observation schedule. *Journal of Autism and Developmental Disorders*, *47*(9), 2770–2782. https://doi.org/10.1007/s10803-017-3176-3

Harry, B., & Klingner, J. K. (2006). *Why are So Many Minority Students in Special Education?: Understanding Race & Disability in Schools*. Teachers College Press.

Hatcher, S. & Waguespack, A. (2004) Academic Accommodations for Students with Disabilities In *Helping Children At home and in School II: Handouts for Education* National Association for School Psychologists Bethesda, MD.

Heaton, R. K. (2000). WCST-64 Computer Version 3 for Windows. Odessa, FL: Psychological Assessment Resources.

Hemdi, A., & Daley, D. (2017). The Effectiveness of a Psychoeducation Intervention delivered via WhatsApp for mothers of children with Autism Spectrum Disorder (ASD) in the Kingdom of Saudi Arabia: A randomized controlled trial. *Child: Care, Health and Development*, *43*(6), 933–941. https://doi.org/10.1111/cch.12520

Hendren, R., Halft, S., Black, J., White, N. C. & Hoeft, F. (2018) Recognizing Psychiatric Disorders Comorbidity with Reading Disorders. *Frontiers in Psychiatry.* 9:101.

Hill, P. (2000). ADHD in adulthood. A guide to current theory, diagnosis, and treatment. by M. Weiss, L. Trokenberg Hechtman, & G. Weiss. Johns Hopkins University Press, Baltimore, MD, 1999. pp. 357. £41.50 (HB). *Journal of Child Psychology and Psychiatry*, *41*(8), 1077–1084. https://doi.org/10.1017/s0021963099296412

Hodge, M. A., Sutherland, R., Jeng, K., Bale, G., Batta, P., Cambridge, A., Detheridge, J., Drevensek, S., Edwards, L., Everett, M., Ganesalingam, K., Geier, P., Kass, C., Mathieson, S., McCabe, M., Micallef, K., Molomby, K., Ong, N., Pfeiffer, S., Pope, S., Silove, N. (2019). Agreement between telehealth and face-to-face assessment of intellectual ability in children with specific learning disorder. *Journal of telemedicine and telecare*, *25*(7), 431–437. https://doi.org/10.1177/1357633X18776095

Hollins, S., & Sinason, V. (2000). Psychotherapy, learning disabilities and trauma: new perspectives. *British Journal of Psychiatry*, *176*(1), 32–36. https://doi.org/10.1192/bjp.176.1.32

Hoofman, J., & Secord, E. (2021). The effect of covid-19 on Education. *Pediatric Clinics of North America*, *68*(5), 1071–1079. https://doi.org/10.1016/j.pcl.2021.05.009

Horacek, H., Ramey, C. T., Campbell, F., Hoffmann, K. P., & Fletcher, R. H. (1987). Predicting School Failure and Assessing Early Intervention with High-Risk Children. *Journal of the American Academy of Child and Adolescent Psychiatry*, *26*(5), 758–763. https://doi.org/10.1097/00004583-198709000-00024

Horn, W. F., Ialongo, N. S., Pascoe, J. M., Greenberg, G., Packard, T., Lopez, M., Wagner, A., & Puttler, L. (1991). Additive effects of psychostimulants, parent training, and self-control therapy with ADHD children. *Journal of the American Academy of Child and Adolescent Psychiatry*, *30*(2), 233–240. https://doi.org/10.1097/00004583-199103000-00011

Horowitz, S. H., Rawe, J., & Whitaker, M. C. (2017). Learning Disabilities; Understanding the 1 in 5. *National Center for Learning Disabilities*. htttps://www.ncld.org/research/state-of-learning-disabilities

Howe, S. M. (2013) Academic Accommodations, social support and academic self-efficacy

Human, M. T., & Teglasi, H. (1994). Parents' satisfaction and compliance with recommendations following psychoeducational assessment of children. *Journal of School Psychology*, *31*(4), 449–464.

Ialongo, N. S., Horn, W. F., Pascoe, J. M., Greenberg, G., Packard, T., Lopez, M., Wagner, A. E., & Puttler, L. I. (1993). The Effects of a Multimodal Intervention with Attention-deficit Hyperactivity Disorder Children: A 9-Month Follow-up. *Journal of the American Academy of Child and Adolescent Psychiatry*, *32*(1), 182–189. https://doi.org/10.1097/00004583-199301000-00026

Ijalba, Elizabeth. (2015). "Understanding Parental Engagement in Hispanic Mothers of Children with Autism Spectrum Disorder: Application of a Process-Model of Cultural Competence." *Journal of Multilingual Education Research*.

International Dyslexia Association. (n.d.). *International Dyslexia Association– . . . until everyone can read!*https://dyslexiaida.org/

Jackson, K. R. & Ferrel, D. R. (2000). Improving recruitment and retention of college students with disabilities. In Hurst, A. (Ed) *The Accessible millennium*, Alodershot, UK: Ashgate Publishing.

Jacobson, R. M, Hanson, W. E. & Zhou, H. (2015). Canadian Psychologists' Test Feedback Training and Practice: A National Survey. *Canadian Psychology, 56*(4), 394–404.

Jenkins, S., Bax, M., Hart, H., (1980) Behavior problems in preschool children. *Journal Child Psychology and Psychiatry.* 21:5–17.

Jensen, C. M., Amdisen, B. L., Jørgensen, K. J., & Arnfred, S. M. H. (2016). Cognitive behavioral therapy for ADHD in adults: systematic review and meta-analyses. *ADHD Attention Deficit and Hyperactivity Disorders*, *8*(1), 3–11. https://doi.org/10.1007/s12402-016-0188-3

Jiao, W. Y., Wang, L. N., Liu, J., Fang, S. F., Jiao, F. Y., Pettoello-Mantovani, M., & Somekh, E. (2020). Behavioral and Emotional Disorders in Children during the COVID-19 Epidemic. *The Journal of pediatrics, 221*, 264–266.e1. https://doi.org/10.1016/j.jpeds.2020.03.013

Jiménez-Muñoz, L., Peñuelas-Calvo, I., Calvo-Rivera, P., Díaz-Oliván, I., Moreno, M., Baca-García, E., & Porras-Segovia, A. (2021). Video games for the treatment of autism spectrum disorder: A systematic review. *Journal of Autism and Developmental Disorders, 52*(1), 169–188. https://doi.org/10.1007/s10803-021-04934-9

Johnson, B. (2005). Psychological Co-Morbidity in Children and Adolescents with Learning Disorders. *Journal of the Indian Association of Child and Adolescent Mental Health* 7:55–59.

Johnson, C. P., & Myers, S. M. (2007). Identification and Evaluation of Children With Autism Spectrum Disorders. *PEDIATRICS, 120*(5), 1183–1215. https://doi.org/10.1542/peds.2007-2361

Jones, J. D. (2002). Plea for a measure of understanding: The importance of intensive psychotherapy in the treatment of children with ADHD. *Psychotherapy: Theory, Research, Practice, Training, 39*(1), 12–20. https://doi.org/10.1037/0033-3204.39.1.12

Judge, S. L. (2000). Computer applications in programs for young children with disabilities: Current status and future directions. *Journal of Special Education Technology, 16*(1), 29–40. https://doi.org/10.1177/016264340101600103

Kalb, L. G., Singh, V., Hong, J. J., Holingue, C., Ludwig, N. N., Pfeiffer, D., Reetzke, R., Gross, A. L., & Landa, R. (2022). Analysis of race and sex bias in the Autism Diagnostic Observation Schedule (ADOS-2). *JAMA Network Open, 5*(4), e229498. https://doi.org/10.1001/jamanetworkopen.2022.9498

Kalvin, C., Jordan, R., Rowley, S., Weis, A., Wood, K. S., Wood, J. J., Ibrahim, K., & Sukhodolsky, D. G. (2021). Conducting CBT for Anxiety in Children with Autism Spectrum Disorder During COVID-19 Pandemic. *Journal of Autism and Developmental Disorders, 51*(11), 4239–4247. https://doi.org/10.1007/s10803-020-04845-1

Kane, J. & Gill, R. P. (1972) Implications of the Purdue Pegboard as a screening device. *Journal of Learning Disabilities*, 547, 36–40.

Kanner, L. (1971) Follow up study of eleven autistic children originally reported in 1943. Journal of Autism and Childhood Schizophrenia, 1, 119–145.

Katz, L. J., Goldstein, G., & Beers, S. R. (2001). Learning disabilities in older adolescents and adults. *Critical Issues in Neuropsychology*. https://doi.org/10.1007/b108001

Keith, R. W. (2000). *SCAN-C, Tests for Auditory Processing Disorders in Children*. San Antonio, TX. The Psychological Corporation.

Kelly, K. & Ramundo, P. (2006) *You Mean I'm Not Stupid, Lazy or Crazy? The classic self-help book for adults with Attention Deficit Disorder.* Simon and Schuster, New York.

Kinnaer, M., Baumers, S., & Heylighen, A. (2015). Autism-friendly architecture from the outside in and the inside out: an explorative study based on autobiographies of autistic people. *Journal of Housing and the Built Environment, 31*(2), 179–195. https://doi.org/10.1007/s10901-015-9451-8

Klingner, J. K., & Harry, B. (2006). The special education referral and decision-making process for English language learners: Child study team meetings and placement conferences. *Teachers College Record: The Voice of Scholarship in Education*, *108*(11), 2247–2281. https://doi.org/10.1111/j.1467-9620.2006.00781.x

Klingner, J. K., Ahwee, S., Pilonieta, P., & Menendez, R. (2003). Barriers and facilitators in scaling up research-based practices. *Exceptional Children*, *69*(4), 411–429. https://doi.org/10.1177/001440290306900402

Koenig, K. (2012). *Practical social skills for autism spectrum disorders; designing child-specific interventions*. New York: W.W. Norton.

Koenig, K., & Levine, M. (2010). Psychotherapy for individuals with autism spectrum disorders. *Journal of Contemporary Psychotherapy*, *41*(1), 29–36. https://doi.org/10.1007/s10879-010-9158-9

Kohut, H. (1971). *The analysis of the self: a systematic approach to the psychoanalytic treatment of narcissistic personality disorders*. University Of Chicago Press.

Kohut, H., & Strozier, C. B. (1985). *Self psychology and the humanities: reflections on a new psychoanalytic approach*. New York: W.W. Norton.

Kopelman-Rubin, D., Klomek, A. B., Al-Yagon, M., Musfon, L., Apter, A., & Mikulincer, M. (2012). Psychological intervention for adolescents diagnosed with learning disorders -"I can succeed" (ICS): Treatment model, feasibility, and acceptability. *International Journal for Research in Learning Disabilities, 1*(1), 37–54.

Korpa, T., Pappa, T., Chouliaras, G., Sfinari, A., Eleftheriades, A., Katsounas, M., Kanaka-Gantenbein, C., & Pervanidou, P. (2021). Daily Behaviors, Worries and Emotions in Children and Adolescents with ADHD and Learning Difficulties during the COVID-19 Pandemic. *Children (Basel, Switzerland)*, *8*(11), 995. https://doi.org/10.3390/children8110995

Kurth, J. A., & Mastergeorge, A. M. (2010). Academic and cognitive profiles of students with autism: Implications for classroom practice and placement. *International Journal of Special Education*, *25*(2).

Lai, M. C., Lombardo, M. V., Auyeung, B., Chakrabarti, B., & Baron-Cohen, S. (2015). Sex/gender differences and autism: setting the scene for future research. *Journal of the American Academy of Child and Adolescent Psychiatry*, *54*(1), 11–24. https://doi.org/10.1016/j.jaac.2014.10.003

Lee, J. (2020) Mental health effects of school closures during COVID-19. *Lancet Child Adolescent Health* 4 (6) 421

Leung, C., Tsang, S., Ng, G. S., & Choi, S. Y. (2016). Efficacy of parent–child interaction therapy with Chinese ADHD children. *Research on Social Work Practice*, *27*(1), 36–47. https://doi.org/10.1177/1049731516643837

Leung, R. C., Vogan, V. M., Powell, T. L., Anagnostou, E., & Taylor, M. J. (2015). The role of executive functions in social impairment in Autism Spectrum Disorder. *Child Neuropsychology*, *22*(3), 336–344. https://doi.org/10.1080/09297049.2015.1005066

Levy-Warren, M. H. (2017). Growing Up With Hatred: A Psychoanalytic Developmental Perspective. *Journal of Infant, Child, and Adolescent Psychotherapy*, *16*(3), 209–218. https://doi.org/10.1080/15289168.2017.1341240

Lipinski, S., Blanke, E. S., Suenkel, U., & Dziobek, I. (2018). Outpatient psychotherapy for adults with high-functioning autism spectrum condition: Utilization, treatment satisfaction, and preferred modifications. *Journal of Autism and Developmental Disorders, 49*(3), 1154–1168. https://doi.org/10.1007/s10803-018-3797-1

Lipinski, S., Boegl, K., Blanke, E. S., Suenkel, U., & Dziobek, I. (2021). A blind spot in mental healthcare? Psychotherapists lack education and expertise for the support of adults on the autism spectrum. *Autism*, 136236132110579. https://doi.org/10.1177/13623613211057973

Loman, M., Vogt, E., Miller, L., Landsman, R., Duong, P., Kasten, J., DeFrancisco, D., Koop, J., & Heffelfinger, A. (2021). "How to" operate a pediatric neuropsychology practice during the COVID-19 pandemic: Real tips from one practice's experience. *Child neuropsychology: a journal on normal and abnormal development in childhood and adolescence*, *27*(2), 251–279. https://doi.org/10.1080/09297049.2020.1830962

Lovett, B. (2012). Educational accommodations for students with disabilities: Two Equity-related concerns.Frontiers in Education, 6, p. 795266. https\\www.frontiersin.org

Lovett, B. J. & Leja, A. M., (2013). Student's perceptions of testing accommodations: What we know, what we need to know and why it matters. *Journal of Applied School Psychology* 29 (1), 72–89.

Łuszczki, E., Bartosiewicz, A., Pezdan-Śliż, I., Kuchciak, M., Jagielski, P., Oleksy, Ł., Stolarczyk, A., & Dereń, K. (2021). Children's Eating Habits, Physical Activity, Sleep, and Media Usage before and during COVID-19 Pandemic in Poland. *Nutrients*, *13*(7), 2447. https://doi.org/10.3390/nu13072447

Maccini, P., & Hughes, C. A. (2000). Effects of a problem-solving strategy on the introductory algebra performance of Secondary students with learning disabilities. *Learning Disabilities Research and Practice*, *15*(1), 10–21. https://doi.org/10.1207/sldrp1501_2

Magaña, S., Lopez, K., & Machalicek, W. (2015). Parents Taking Action: A Psycho-Educational Intervention for Latino Parents of Children With Autism Spectrum Disorder. *Family Process*, *56*(1), 59–74. https://doi.org/10.1111/famp.12169

Maier, C. A., Riger, D., & Morgan-Sowada, H. (2021). "it's splendid once you grow into it:" client experiences of relational teletherapy in the era of Covid-19. *Journal of Marital and Family Therapy*, *47*(2), 304–319. https://doi.org/10.1111/jmft.12508

Mancini, P. & Gagnon, J. C. (2006). Mathematics instruction and assessment accommodations by secondary special and general educators. *Exceptional Children*, 72, 217–234.

Mandell, D. S., Ittenbach, R. F., Levy, S. E., & Pinto-Martin, J. (2006). Disparities in diagnoses received prior to a diagnosis of autism spectrum disorder. *Journal of Autism and Developmental Disorders*, *37*(9), 1795–1802. https://doi.org/10.1007/s10803-006-0314-8

Mandell, D. S., Listerud, J., Levy, S. E., & Pinto-Martin, J. (2002). Race differences in the age at diagnosis among Medicaid-Eligible Children with autism. *Journal of the American Academy of Child and Adolescent Psychiatry*, *41*(12), 1447–1453. https://doi.org/10.1097/00004583-200212000-00016

Manganello, R. E. (1992). Psychosocial Problems Among Learning Disabled College Students. *Research and Teaching in Developmental Education*, *9*(1), 67–78. http://www.jstor.org/stable/42801849

Mangrum, C. T., & Strichart, S. S. (1984). *College and the Learning Disabled Student*. Orlando, FL: Grune & Stratton.

Margalit, M. (1995). Social Skills Learning for students with learning disabilities and students with behaviour disorders. *Educational Psychology*, *15*(4), 445–456. https://doi.org/10.1080/0144341950150407

Margalit, M. & Shulman, S. (1986). Autonomy perceptions and anxiety expressions of learning diesabled adolescents. *Journal of Learning Disabilities*, 19, 291–293.

Markowitz, J. C., Milrod, B., Heckman, T. G., Bergman, M., Amsalem, D., Zalman, H., Ballas, T., & Neria, Y. (2021). Psychotherapy at a Distance. *The American journal of psychiatry*, *178*(3), 240–246. https://doi.org/10.1176/appi.ajp.2020.20050557

Markram, K. & Markram, H. (2010). The intense world theory: A unifying theory of the neurobiology of autism. Front. Hum. Neurosci. 4:224.

Maroda, K. J. (1999). Creating an intersubjective context for self-disclosure. *Smith College Studies in Social Work, 69*(2), 474–489. https://doi.org/10.1080/00377319909517566

Marshak, L., Van Wieren, T., Fereel, D. R., Swiss, L., & Dugan, C. (2010). Exploring barriers to college student use of disability services and accomodations. *Journal of Postsecondary Education and Disability* 22 (3), 151–165.

Martin, C. S., Romig, C. J., & Kirisci, L. (2000). DSM-IV learning disorders in 10- to 12-year-old boys with and without a parental history of substance use disorders. *Prevention Science*. https://doi.org/10.1023/a:1010042231697 Prev Sci. 2000 Jun;1(2):107–13. doi: 10.1023/a:1010042231697. PMID: 11521959.

Martin, S. & Zirkel, P. (2011). Identification disputes for students with attention deficit hyperactivity disorder: An analysis of the case law. *School Psychology Review* 40 (3) 405–422.

Mascheretti, S., Trezzi, V., Giorda, R., Boivin, M., Plourde, V., & Vitaro, F. (2017). Complex effects of dyslexia risk factors account for ADHD traits: evidence from two independent samples. *Journal of Child Psychology and Psychiatry* 58(1): 75–82.

Masse, J. J., McNeil, C. B., Wagner, S. M., & Chorney, D. B. (2007). Parent-child interaction therapy and high functioning autism: A conceptual overview. *Journal of Early and Intensive Behavior Intervention*, *4*(4), 714–735. https://doi.org/10.1037/h0100402

Masten, A. S., Roisman, G. I., Long, J. D., Burt, K. B., Obradović, J., Riley, J. R., Boelcke-Stennes, K., & Tellegen, A. (2005). Developmental cascades: linking academic achievement and externalizing and internalizing symptoms over 20 years. *Developmental psychology*, *41*(5), 733–746. https://doi.org/10.1037/0012-1649.41.5.733

Mather, N. & Wendling, N. J. (2011) *Essentials of Dyslexia Assessment and Intervention*. Hoboken, NJ: John Wiley.

Matson, J. L., & Goldin, R. L. (2013). Comorbidity and autism: Trends, topics and future directions. *Research in Autism Spectrum Disorders*, *7*(10), 1228–1233. https://doi.org/10.1016/j.rasd.2013.07.003

Matson, M. L., Mahan, S., & Matson, J. L. (2009). Parent training: A review of methods for children with autism spectrum disorders. *Research in Autism Spectrum Disorders*, *3*(4), 868–875. https://doi.org/10.1016/j.rasd.2009.02.003

McCarthy, J. & Conway, F. (2011). Attention Deficit Hyperactivity Disorder in Children and the Psychoanalytic Process. *Journal of Infant, Child and Adolescent Psychotherapy,* 10 (1), pp. 1–4.

McConachie, H., McLaughlin, E., Grahame, V., Taylor, H., Honey, E., Tavernor, L., Rodgers, J., Freeston, M., Hemm, C., Steen, N., & Le Couteur, A. (2014). Group therapy for anxiety in children with autism spectrum disorder. *Autism; the international journal of research and practice*, *18*(6), 723–732. https://doi.org/10.1177/1362361313488839

McCullough A. (2001). Viability and effectiveness of teletherapy for pre-school children with special needs. *International journal of language & communication disorders*, *36 Suppl*, 321–326. https://doi.org/10.3109/13682820109177905

McCusker, E. (1994). The American Disability Act: Potential for expanding the Scope of reasonable academic accommodations. *J.C & UL,* 21, 619.

Meersand, P. (2011). Psychological testing and the analytically trained child psychologist. *Psychoanalytic Psychology*, *28*(1), 117.

Menaker, E. (1990). Transference, Countertransference, and therapeutic efficacy in relation to Self-Disclosure by the analyst. *Self-Disclosure in the Therapeutic Relationship*, 103–115. https://doi.org/10.1007/978-1-4899-3582-3_8

Menghini, D., Finzi, A., Benassi, M., Bolzani, R., Facoetti, A., Giovagnoli, S., Ruffino, M., & Vicari, S. (2010). Different underlying neurocognitive deficits in developmental dyslexia: A comparative study. *Neuropsychologia*, *48*(4), 863–872. https://doi.org/10.1016/j.neuropsychologia.2009.11.003

Mervosh, S. (2022). The pandemic erased two decades of progress in math and reading. *The New York Times.*

Meyer, G. J., Finn, S. E., Eyde, L. D., Kay, G. G., Moreland, K. L., Dies, R. R., & Reed, G. M. (2001). Psychological testing and psychological assessment: A review of evidence and issues. *American psychologist*, *56*(2), 128.

Meyer, G. J., Viglione, D. J., Mihur, J. L., Erard, R. E. & Erdag, P. (2011). *Rorschach Performance Assessment System: Admission, Coding, Interpretation and Technical Manual.* Toledo, Ohio, RAPS, LLC.

Milsom, A. & Hartley, M. T. (2005). Assisting students with learning disabilities transitioning to college: What school counselors should know. *Professional School Counseling.*8, 436–441.

Milsom, A., Akos, P., & Thompson, M. (2004). A Psychoeducational Group Approach to Postsecondary Transition Planning for Students with Learning Disabilities. *The Journal for Specialists in Group Work*, *29*(4), 395–411. https://doi.org/10.1080/01933920490516170

Mindt, M. R., Arentoft, A., Germano, K. K., D'Aquila, E., Scheiner, D., Pizzirusso, M., Gollan, T. H. (2008). Neuropsychological, Cognitive, and Theoretical Considerations for Evaluation of Bilingual Individuals. *Neuropsychology Review*, *18*(3), 255–268. http://doi.org/10.1007/s11065-008-9069-7

Miranda, A., & Jess Presentacin, M. (2000). Efficacy of Cognitive-Behavioral therapy in the treatment of children with adhd, with and without aggressiveness. *Psychology in the Schools*, *37*(2), 169–182. https://doi.org/3.0.co;2-8”>10.1002/(sici)1520-6807(200003)37:2<169::aid-pits8>3.0.co;2-8

Mishna, F., Kaiman, J., Little, S., & Tarshis, E. (1994). Group therapy with adolescents who have learning disabilities and social/emotional problems. *Journal of Child and Adolescent Group Therapy*, *4*(2), 117–131. https://doi.org/10.1007/bf02548484

Mitchell, J. T., Zylowska, L., & Kollins, S. H. (2015). Mindfulness meditation training for attention-deficit/hyperactivity disorder in adulthood: Current empirical support, treatment overview, and future directions. *Cognitive and Behavioral Practice*, *22*(2), 172–191. https://doi.org/10.1016/j.cbpra.2014.10.002

Mitchell, S. A. (1988). *Relational concepts in psychoanalysis: An integration.* Harvard University Press.

Montoya, A., Colom, F., & Ferrin, M. (2011). Is psychoeducation for parents and teachers of children and adolescents with ADHD efficacious? A systematic literature review. *European Psychiatry*, *26*(3), 166–175. https://doi.org/10.1016/j.eurpsy.2010.10.005

Moore, J. R., Hanson, W. R., & Maxey, E. C. (2020). Disability Inclusion: Catalyst to adaptive organizations. *Industrial and Organizational Psychology.* 14, 76–80

More, C. (2008). Digital stories targeting social skills for children with disabilities. *Intervention in School and Clinic*, *43*(3), 168–177. https://doi.org/10.1177/1053451207312919

Mufson, L., Moreau, D., Weissman, M. M., Wickramaratne, P., Martin, J., & Samoilov, A. (1994). Modification of interpersonal psychotherapy with depressed adolescents (IPT-A): phase I and II studies. *Journal of the American Academy of Child and Adolescent Psychiatry*, *33*(5), 695–705. https://doi.org/10.1097/00004583-199406000-00011

Murray, H. A. (1943). *Thematic Apperception Test.* Cambridge, MA: Harvard University Press.

Narvaez, R. A. (2022). Benefits and challenges of telepsychiatry services in Southeast Asian nations during the COVID-19 ERA: An integrative review. *Asian Journal of Psychiatry*, *73*, 103114. https://doi.org/10.1016/j.ajp.2022.103114

Nigg, J. T. (2012). Future directions in ADHD etiology research. *Journal of Clinical Child & Adolescent Psychology*, *41*(4), 524–533. https://doi.org/10.1080/15374416.2012.686870

Norbury, C., Gooch, D., Wray, C., Baird, G., Charman, T., Simonoff, E., Vamvakas, G., & Pickles, A. (2016). The impact of nonverbal ability on prevalence and clinical presentation of language disorder: evidence from a population study. *Journal of Child Psychology and Psychiatry*, *57*(11), 1247–1257. https://doi.org/10.1111/jcpp.12573

Norwich, B. (2008). Special schools: What future for special schools and inclusion? conceptual and professional perspectives. *British Journal of Special Education*, *35*(3), 136–143. https://doi.org/10.1111/j.1467-8578.2008.00387.x

Nussey, C., Pistrang, N., & Murphy, T. (2013). How does psychoeducation help? A review of the effects of providing information about Tourette syndrome and attention-deficit/hyperactivity disorder. *Child: Care, Health and Development*, *39*(5), 617–627. https://doi.org/10.1111/cch.12039

O'Driscoll, D. (2014). Shame and its role in the lives of people with learning disabilities. *Learning Disability Practice*. 21 (2), 14.

Ogilvy, C. M. (1994). Social Skills Training with Children and Adolescents: a review of the evidence on effectiveness. *Educational Psychology*, *14*(1), 73–83. https://doi.org/10.1080/0144341940140105

Oomen, D., Nijhof, A. D., & Wiersema, J. R. (2021). The psychological impact of the COVID-19 pandemic on adults with autism: A survey study across three countries. *Molecular Autism*, *12*(1). https://doi.org/10.1186/s13229-021-00424-y

Oono, I. P., Honey, E. J., & McConachie, H. (2013). Parent-mediated early intervention for young children with autism spectrum disorders (ASD). *Cochrane Database of Systematic Reviews*. https://doi.org/10.1002/14651858.cd009774.pub2

Orenstein, M. (2000). Picking up the clues: Understanding undiagnosed learning disabilities,

Orenstein, M. (2007). *Smart but stuck: How resilience frees imprisoned intelligence from learning Disabilities*. Philadelphia: Haworth Press.

Osman, B. (2000). Learning Disabilities and the Risk of Psychiatric Disorders in Children and Adolescents in *Learning Disabilities: Implications for Psychiatric Treatment.* L. Greenhill, Ed. Review of Psychiatry, Volume 19 (5). American Psychiatric Press, Washington, DC.

PACER Center (2001) ACTion sheet: PHP-C49, Minneapolis, MN www.PACER.org

Palombo, J. (2001). *Learning Disorders & Disorders of the Self in Children & Adolescents*. W.W. Norton: New York.

Papanastasiou F. (2018) The psychological implication of learning disabilities. *Acta Psychopathology. Vol.* 4.

Parellada, M., Penzol, M. J., Pina, L., Moreno, C., González-Vioque, E., Zalsman, G., & Arango, C. (2014). The Neurobiology of Autism Spectrum Disorders. *European Psychiatry*, *29*(1), 11–19. https://doi.org/10.1016/j.eurpsy.2013.02.005

Parker, D. R., Field, S., Sawilowsky, S, Rolands, L. (2011). An examination of the effects of ADHD coaching on university students' executive functioning. *Journal of PostSecondary Education and Disability* 24 (2), 115–132.

Parsons, M. W., Gardner, M. M., Sherman, J. C., Pasquariello, K., Grieco, J. A., Kay, C. D., Pollak, L. E., Morgan, A. K., Carlson-Emerton, B., Seligsohn, K., Davidsdottir, S., Pulsifer, M. B., Zarrella, G. V., Burstein, S. M., & Mancuso, S. M. (2022). Feasibility and Acceptance of Direct-to-Home Tele-neuropsychology Services during the COVID-19 Pandemic. *Journal of the International Neuropsychological Society; JINS*, *28*(2), 210–215. https://doi.org/10.1017/S1355617721000436

Patra, S., Arun, P., & Chavan, B. (2015). Impact of psychoeducation intervention module on parents of children with autism spectrum disorders: A preliminary study. *Journal of Neurosciences in Rural Practice*, *6*(4), 529. https://doi.org/10.4103/0976-3147.165422

Pelham, W. E., & Fabiano, G. A. (2008). Evidence-based psychosocial treatments for attention-deficit/hyperactivity disorder. *Journal of Clinical Child & Adolescent Psychology*, *37*(1), 184–214. https://doi.org/10.1080/15374410701818681

Peluso, M. A., & Guerra de Andrade, L. H. (2005). Physical activity and mental health: the association between exercise and mood. *Clinics (Sao Paulo, Brazil)*, *60*(1), 61–70. https://doi.org/10.1590/s1807-59322005000100012

Pennington, B. F., & Bishop, D. V. M. (2009). Relations among speech, language, and reading disorders. *Annual Review of Psychology*, *60*(1), 283–306. https://doi.org/10.1146/annurev.psych.60.110707.163548

Phillips, S. E. (1994). High stakes testing accommodations: Validity versus disabled rights. *Applied Measures Education* 7 (2) 93–120.

Pintrich, P. R. (2002). The role of metacognitive knowledge in learning, teaching, and assessing. *Theory Into Practice*, *41*(4), 219–225. https://doi.org/10.1207/s15430421tip4104_3

Plavnick, J. B., Bak, M. Y. S., Avendaño, S. M., Dueñas, A. D., Brodhead, M. T., & Sipila, E. S. (2020). Implementing early intensive behavioral intervention in community settings. *Autism*, *24*(7), 1913–1916. https://doi.org/10.1177/1362361320919243

Poelmans, G., Buitelaar, J. K., Pauls, D. L., & Franke, B. (2010). A theoretical molecular network for dyslexia: integrating available genetic findings. *Molecular Psychiatry*, *16*(4), 365–382. https://doi.org/10.1038/mp.2010.105

Pollak, J. M. (1988). The feedback process with parents in child and adolescent psychological assessment. *Psychology in the Schools*.

Postorino, V., Sharp, W. G., McCracken, C. E., Bearss, K., Burrell, T. L., Evans, A. N., & Scahill, L. (2017). A Systematic Review and Meta-analysis of Parent Training for Disruptive Behavior in Children with Autism Spectrum Disorder. *Clinical Child and Family Psychology Review*, *20*(4), 391–402. https://doi.org/10.1007/s10567-017-0237-2

Prelock, P. A., Beatson, J., Bitner, B., Broder, C., & Ducker, A. (2003). Interdisciplinary Assessment of Young Children With Autism Spectrum Disorder. *Language, speech, and hearing services in schools*, *34*(3), 194–202. https://doi.org/10.1044/0161-1461(2003/016)Jul 1;34(3):194–202. doi: 10.1044/0161-1461(2003/016). PMID: 27764321.

Preston, A. I. (2016). *Effects of Singapore model method with explicit instruction on math problem solving skills of students at risk for or identified with learning disabilities* (Order No. 10139928). Available from ProQuest Dissertations & Theses A&I; ProQuest Dissertations & Theses Global; ProQuest One Academic. (1805310285). https://colorado.idm.oclc.org/login?url=https://www.proquest.com/dissertations-theses/effects-singapore-model-method-with-explicit/docview/1805310285/se-2

Pritchard, A. E., Koniakin, T., Carey, L., Bellows, A., Jacobson, L., & Mahone, M. (2016). Academic testing accommodations for ADHD: Do they help? *Learning Disabilities* 21 (2) 67–78.

Prizant, B. M., Audet, L. R., Burke, G. M., Hummel, L. J., Maher, S. R., Thedore, G. (1990). Communication Disorders and Emotional/Behavioral Disorders in Children and Adolescents. *Journal of Speech and Hearing Disorders*. 55 (2) 179–192.

Putnam, J. W., Spiegel, A. N., & Bruininks, R. H. (1995). Future directions in education and inclusion of students with disabilities: A delphi investigation. *Exceptional Children*, *61*(6), 553–576. https://doi.org/10.1177/001440299506100605

Raizada, R. D., & Kishiyama, M. M. (2010). Effects of socioeconomic status on brain development, and how cognitive neuroscience may contribute to levelling the playing field. *Frontiers in human neuroscience*, *4*, 3. https://doi.org/10.3389/neuro.09.003.2010

Ramsay, J. R., & Rostain, A. L. (2007). Psychosocial treatments for attention-deficit/hyperactivity disorder in adults: Current evidence and future directions. *Professional Psychology: Research and Practice*, *38*(4), 338–346. https://doi.org/10.1037/0735-7028.38.4.338

Ratey, J. J., Greenberg, M. S., Bemporad, J. R., & Lindem, K. (1992). Unrecognized Attention-Deficit hyperactivity Disorder in adults presenting for outpatient psychotherapy. *Journal of Child and Adolescent Psychopharmacology*, *2*(4), 267–275. https://doi.org/10.1089/cap.1992.2.267

Reese, R. J., Conoley, C. W., & Brossart, D. F. (2002). Effectiveness of telephone counseling: A field-based investigation. *Journal of Counseling Psychology, 49*(2), 233–242.

Reichow, B. (2011). Overview of meta-analyses on early intensive behavioral intervention for young children with autism spectrum disorders. *Journal of Autism and Developmental Disorders*, *42*(4), 512–520. https://doi.org/10.1007/s10803-011-1218-9

Reid, D., & Knight, M. (2006). Disability Justifies Exclusion of Minority Students: A Critical History Grounded in Disability Studies. *Educational Researcher*, *35*(6), 18–23. https://doi.org/10.3102/0013189x035006018

Resources for Language-Based Learning Differences. Verticy Learning (2009)

Reynolds, C. R. & Kamphaus, R. W. (2020). Behavior Assessment for Children: third edition (BASC-3) Bloomington, MN: Pearson.

Richman, E., Randemacher, G. N. & Maitland, T. L. (2014). Coaching and college success. *Journal of PostSecondary Education and Disability* 27 (1) 35–50.

Riglin, L., Leppert, B., Langley, K., Thapar, A., O'Donovan, M., Smith, G., Stergiakouli, E., Tilling, K, Thapar, A. (2020) Investigating attention deficit hyperactivity disorder and autism spectrum disorder traits in the general population: What happens in adult life? *Journal of Child Psychology and Psychiatry.* Volume 62, 4:449–457.

Ritchey, K.D & Goeke, J. L. (2006) Orton-Gillingham and Orton-Gillingham based reading intervention: A review of the literature. *The Journal of Special Education.* 40 (3), 171–183.

of the literature. *The Journal of Special Education.* 40 (3), 171–183.

Rivera Mindt, Monica, et al. "Neuropsychological, Cognitive, and Theoretical Considerations for Evaluation of Bilingual Individuals." *Neuropsychology Review*, vol. 18, no. 3, Sept. 2008, pp. 255–268, 10.1007/s11065-008-9069-7.

Roman-Urrestarazu, Andres, et al. "Association of Race/Ethnicity and Social Disadvantage with Autism Prevalence in 7 Million School Children in England." *JAMA Pediatrics*, vol. 175, no. 6, 29 Mar. 2021, p. e210054, 10.1001/jamapediatrics.2021.0054.

Rorschach, H (1921) *Psychodiagnostik*. Bern:Bircher (Transl. Hans Huber Verlag, 1942)

Rothstein, A. A., & Glenn, J. (2001). Review of Learning Disabilities and Psychic Conflict: A Psychoanalytic Casebook. *Psychoanalytic Psychology*, *18*(3), 623–626. https://doi.org/10.1037/0736-9735.18.3.623

Royer, J. M. & Randall, J. (2012). Testing Accommodations for Students with Disabilities in *APA Educational Psychological Handbook: Volume 3.*

Rumsey, J. M. & Hamburger, S. D. (1990) Neuropsychological Divergence of high-level Autism and Severe Dyslexia. Journal of Autism and Developmental Disorders. 20, 155–168.

Russell, T. L. (2001). *The no significant difference phenomenon: A comparative research annotated bibliography on technology for distance education; as reported in 355 research reports, summaries and papers*. Raleigh, N.C: IDECC.

Ryan, A. G. & Heikkila, M. K. (1988). Learning Disabilities in Higher Education: Misconceptions, *Academic Therapy* 24(2) 177–192.

Rycroft, C. (1972). *Critical dictionary of psychoanalysis.* Pennsylvania: Penn State University Press

Sabin, J. A., & Greenwald, A. G. (2012). The influence of implicit bias on treatment recommendations for 4 common pediatric conditions: pain, urinary tract infection, attention deficit hyperactivity disorder, and asthma. *American Journal of Public Health*, *102*(5), 988–995. https://doi.org/10.2105/ajph.2011.300621

Sahoo, M. K., Biswas, H., & Padhy, S. K. (2015). Psychological Co-morbidity in Children with Specific Learning Disorders. *Journal of family medicine and primary care*, *4*(1), 21–25. https://doi.org/10.4103/2249-4863.152243

Saifi, S. & Mehmood, T. (2011). Effects of socio-economic status on students achievement. *International Journal of Social Sciences and Education*, 1(2), 119–128

Salomonsson, B. (2006). The impact of words on children with ADHD and DAMP Consequences for psychoanalytic technique. *The International Journal of Psychoanalysis*, *87*(4), 1029–1047. https://doi.org/10.1516/eyq4-21hh-1kqj-2wme

Salomonsson, B. (2017). Interpreting the inner world of ADHD children: psychoanalytic perspectives. *International Journal of Qualitative Studies on Health and Well-Being*, *12* (supl), 1298269. https://doi.org/10.1080/17482631.2017.1298269

Sandler, A. D. (1995). Attention deficits and neurodevelopmental variation in older adolescents and adults. *A comprehensive guide to attention deficit disorder in adults: research, diagnosis treatment*, 58–73.

Sarrett, J. C. (2017). Autism and Accommodations in Higher Education: Insights from the Autism Community. *Journal of Autism and Developmental Disorders*, *48*(3), 679–693. https://doi.org/10.1007/s10803-017-3353-4

Satterly, B. A. (2006). Therapist Self-Disclosure from a Gay Male Perspective. *Families in Society, 87*(2), 240–247. https://doi.org/10.1606/1044-3894.3517

Schanen, N. C. (2006). Epigenetics of autism spectrum disorders. *Human Molecular Genetics*, *15*(suppl_2). https://doi.org/10.1093/hmg/ddl213

Schnittker, J. (2003). Misgivings of medicine?: African Americans' skepticism of psychiatric medication. *Journal of Health and Social Behavior*, *44*(4), 506. https://doi.org/10.2307/1519796

Schreibman L. (2000). Intensive behavioral/psychoeducational treatments for autism: research needs and future directions. *Journal of autism and developmental disorders*, *30*(5), 373–378. https://doi.org/10.1023/a:1005535120023

Schultz, B. K., Evans, S. W., Langberg, J. M., & Schoemann, A. M. (2017). Outcomes for adolescents who comply with long-term psychosocial treatment for ADHD. *Journal of Consulting and Clinical Psychology*, *85*(3), 250–261. https://doi.org/10.1037/ccp0000172

Sciberras, E., Patel, P., Stokes, M. A., Coghill, D., Middeldorp, C. M., Bellgrove, M. A., Becker, S. P., Efron, D., Stringaris, A., Faraone, S. V., Bellows, S. T., Quach, J., Banaschewski, T., McGillivray, J., Hutchinson, D., Silk, T. J., Melvin, G., Wood, A. G., Jackson, A., Loram, G., Westrupp, E. (2022). Physical Health, Media Use, and Mental Health in Children and Adolescents With ADHD During the COVID-19 Pandemic in Australia. *Journal of attention disorders,* 26(4), 549–562. https://doi.org/10.1177/1087054720978549

Scott, B. J. & Vitale, M. R. (2003). Teaching the writing process to students with learning disabilities: Intervention in school and clinic 38 (4) 210–224.

Seelig, S (1987). A College Guide for LD Service providers. Long Island University.

Sehon, C. (2015). Teleanalysis and teletherapy for children and adolescents?. In J. Scharff (Ed.), *Psychoanalysis Online 2* (pp. 36–60). London: Routledge.

Seligman, M. (1975). *Helplessness, On Depression, Development and Death,* Freeman, CA.

Semel E., Wiig E., Secord,W.,(2013). *The Clinical Evaluation of Language Fundamentals–Fifth Edition* (CELF-5) Bloomington, MN;NCS, Pearson

Serlachius, A., Badawy, S. M., & Thabrew, H. (2020). Psychosocial Challenges and Opportunities for Youth With Chronic Health Conditions During the COVID-19 Pandemic. *JMIR pediatrics and parenting*, *3*(2), e23057. https://doi.org/10.2196/23057

Shah, R. (1995). *The silent minority: Children with Disabilities in Asian Families.* National Childrens Bureau.

Sharfstein, J. M., & Morphew, C. C. (2020). The Urgency and Challenge of Opening K–12 Schools in the Fall of 2020. *JAMA*, *324*(2), 133–134. https://doi.org/10.1001/jama.2020.10175

Sharma, D., & Bhaskar, S. (2020). Addressing the Covid-19 Burden on Medical Education and Training: The Role of Telemedicine and Tele-Education During and Beyond the Pandemic. *Frontiers in public health*, *8*, 589669. https://doi.org/10.3389/fpubh.2020.589669

Shaw, P., Lerch, J. P., Greenstein, D., Sharp, W., Clasen, L. S., Evans, A. C., Giedd, J. N., Castellanos, F. X., & Rapoport, J. L. (2006). Longitudinal mapping of cortical thickness and clinical outcome in children and adolescents with Attention-Deficit/Hyperactivity Disorder. *Archives of General Psychiatry*, *63*(5), 540. https://doi.org/10.1001/archpsyc.63.5.540

Shaw, M., Hodgkins, P., Caci, H., Young, S., Kahle, J., Woods, A. G., & Arnold, L. E. (2012). A systematic review and analysis of long-term outcomes in attention deficit hyperactivity disorder: effects of treatment and non-treatment. *BMC Medicine*, *10*(1). https://doi.org/10.1186/1741-7015-10-99

Shaywitz, B. E. & Shaywitz, B. A. (2005) Dyslexia (specific learning disability). *Biological Psychiatry,* 52 (2), 1301–1309.

Shaywitz, Sally E. *Overcoming Dyslexia; A New and Complete Science-Based Program for Reading Problems at Any Level*. New York: A.A. Knopf, 2003.

Shessel, I. & Reiff, H. B. (1999) Experiences of Adults with Learning Disabilities: Positive and Negative Impacts and Outcomes. *Learning Disability Quarterly.* 22(4), 305–316.

Shi, Y., Guevara, L. R. H., Dykhoff, H. J., Sangaralingham, L. R., Phelan, S., Zaccariello, M. J., & Warner, D. O. (2021). Racial disparities in diagnosis of Attention-Deficit/Hyperactivity Disorder in a US national birth cohort. *JAMA Network Open*, *4*(3), e210321. https://doi.org/10.1001/jamanetworkopen.2021.0321

Shifrer, D., Muller, C., & Callahan, R. M. (2011). Disproportionality and learning disabilities: parsing apart race, socioeconomic status, and language. *Journal of Learning Disabilities*, *44*(3), 246–257. https://doi.org/10.1177/0022219410374236

Shogren, K. A., Palmer, S. B., Wehmeyer, M. L., Williams-Diehm, K. & Little, T. D. (2012). Effect of intervention with the self-determined learning model of instruction on access and goal attainment. *Remedial and Special Education.*33 (5) 320–3330.

Shonkoff, J. P., & Phillips, D. (2000). From neurons to neighborhoods. In *National Academies Press eBooks*. https://doi.org/10.17226/9824

Sibley, M. H., Ortiz, M., Gaias, L. M., Reyes, R., Joshi, M., Alexander, D., & Graziano, P. (2021). Top problems of adolescents and young adults with ADHD during the COVID-19 pandemic. *Journal of Psychiatric Research*, *136*, 190–197. https://doi.org/10.1016/j.jpsychires.2021.02.009

Siegel, M. G. (1987). Psychological testing from early childhood through adolescence: a developmental and psychodynamic approach. International Universities Press Inc.

Sikirica, V. E., Flood, N. C., Dietrich, J., Quintero, V., Harpin, P., Hodgkins, K., Skrodzki, K., Beusterien, & Erder, H.M (2015). Unmet needs associated with Attention Deficit Hyperactivity Disorder in eight European countries as reported by caregivers and adolescents: results from qualitative research. *The Patient-Patient Centered Outcomes Research* 8 (3) 269–281.

Silk, J. S., Scott, L. N., Hutchinson, E. A., Lu, C., Sequeira, S. L., McKone, K., Do, Q. B., & Ladouceur, C. D. (2022). Storm Clouds and Silver Linings: Day-to-Day Life in COVID-19 Lockdown and Emotional Health in Adolescent Girls. *Journal of pediatric psychology*, *47*(1), 37–48. https://doi.org/10.1093/jpepsy/jsab107

Silver, L (2006) The misunderstood Child. Understanding and Coping with your child's Learning Disabilities. New York: Three Rivers Press.

Sinason, V. (2002). Some reflections from twenty years of psychoanalytic work with children and adults with a learning disability. *Disability Studies Quarterly*. 22 (3), 38–45

Sinason, V. (2002). *Attachment, Trauma and Multiplicity*. Psychology Press.

Sinha, P., Kjelgard, M., Gandhi, T., Tsourides, K., Cardinaux, A. L., & Pantazi, D.

Sireci, S. G., Scarpati, S. E. & Li, S. (2005). Test accommodations for students with disabilities: An analysis of the interaction hypothesis. *Review of Educational Research, 75 (4) 459–490.*

Sisterhen, D. H. & Gerber, P. J. (1989) Auditory, Visual and Multisensory Nonverbal Social Perception in Adolescents with or without Learning Disabilities. *Journal of Learning Disabilities* 22(4) 245–249.

Slobodin, O., & Masalha, R. (2020). Challenges in ADHD care for ethnic minority children: A review of the current literature. *Transcultural Psychiatry*, *57*(3), 468–483. https://doi.org/10.1177/1363461520902885

Smith, K. A., Gehricke, J., Iadarola, S., Wolfe, A. E., & Kuhlthau, K. (2020). Disparities in service use among Children with Autism: a systematic review. *Pediatrics*, *145*(Supplement_1), S35–S46. https://doi.org/10.1542/peds.2019-1895g

Sniatecki, J. L., Perry, H. B., Snell, L. H. (2015). Faculty Attitudes and Knowledge Regarding College Students with Disabilities. *Journal of Postsecondary Education and Disability.* 28(3), 259–275.

Snowling, M. J., Bishop, D. V. M., & Stothard, S. E. (2000). Is preschool language impairment a risk factor for dyslexia in adolescence? *Journal of Child Psychology and Psychiatry*, *41*(5), 587–600. https://doi.org/10.1111/1469-7610.00651

Sorscher, N. (2020). Achieving "Adulting": Working with Young Adults with Neurocognitive Challenges: A Developmental Model. *Journal of Infant, Child, and Adolescent Psychotherapy*, *19*(1), 71–85. https://doi.org/10.1080/15289168.2020.1717254

Sorscher, N. (2022). Psychotherapy with Patients with Neurocognitive Impairments. *Journal of Infant, Child, and Adolescent Psychotherapy*, *21*(1), 1–18. https://doi.org/10.1080/15289168.2022.2050659

Sowell, E. R., Thompson, P. M., Welcome, S. E., Henkenius, A. L., Toga, A. W., & Peterson, B. S. (2003). Cortical abnormalities in children and adolescents with attention-deficit hyperactivity disorder. *The Lancet*, *362*(9397), 1699–1707. https://doi.org/10.1016/s0140-6736(03)14842-8

Stebbins, M. S., Stormont, M., Lembke, E., Wilson, D. T. & Clippard, D. (2012). Monitoring the effectiveness of the Wilson reading system for students with disabilities: One district's example. *Exceptionality* 20(1) 58–70.

Stevens, J., Harman, J. S., & Kelleher, K. J. (2005). Race/Ethnicity and Insurance Status as Factors Associated with ADHD Treatment Patterns. *Journal of Child and Adolescent Psychopharmacology*, *15*(1), 88–96. https://doi.org/10.1089/cap.2005.15.88

Streoop, J. R. (1935) Studies of interference in serial verbal reactions. *Journal of Experimental Psychology, 18*, 643–662.

Sturrock, A., Chilton, H., Foy, K., Freed, J., Admas, C. (2021) In their own words: The impact of subtle language and communication difficulties as described by autisitic girls and boys without intellectual disability. *Autism.* 13623613211002047

Sue, D. W., & Sue, D. (1999). *Counseling the culturally different: Theory and Practice.*

Sugarman, A. (1981). The diagnostic use of countertransference reactions in psychological testing. *Bulletin of the Menninger Clinic*, *45*(6), 473.

Sukhodolsky, D. G., Bloch, M. H., Panza, K. E., & Reichow, B. (2013). Cognitive-Behavioral Therapy for Anxiety in Children With High-Functioning Autism: A Meta-analysis. *PEDIATRICS*, *132*(5), e1341–e1350. https://doi.org/10.1542/peds.2013-1193

Sundheim, S., & Voeller, K. (2004). Psychiatric Implications of Language Disorders and Learning Disabilities: Risks and Management. *Journal of Child Neurology.* Volume 19, Number 10.

Suvarna Latha, R., Karalam, S., Mathew, J., Joseph, S. (2022). A Scoping Review of Formal Care to Children with Special Needs during the Covid-19 Pandemic. *International Journal of Special Education, 37*(1), 1–14

Svetaz, M. V., Ireland, M., Blum, R. (2000). Adolescents with learning disabilities: risk and protective factors associated with emotional well being: findings from the National Longitudinal Study of Adolescent Health. *Journal of Adolescent Health* Volume 27, Issue 5, 340–348.

Sweener, K., Kundert, D., May, D., & Quinn, K. (2013). Comfort with accommodations at the community college level. *Journal of Developmental Education,* 25 (3), 12–18.

Tajik-Parvinchi, D., Farmus, L., Modica, P. T., Cribbie, R. A., & Weiss, J. A. (2021). The role of cognitive control and emotion regulation in predicting mental health problems in children with neurodevelopmental disorders. *Child Care Health and Development*, *47*(5), 608–617. https://doi.org/10.1111/cch.12868

Tavani, C. M. (2004). *The impact of testing accommodations on students with learning disabilities: An investigation of the 2000 NAEP mathematics assessment* (Order No. 3137495). Available from ProQuest Dissertations & Theses A&I; ProQuest Dissertations & Theses Global; ProQuest One Academic. (305182301). https://colorado.idm.oclc.org/login?url=https://www.proquest.com/dissertations-theses/impact-testing-accommodations-on-students-with/docview/305182301/se-2

Thambirajah, M. S. and Ramanujan, L. L. (2016) Essentials of Learning Disabilities and Other Developmental Disorders, Sage Publications, India.

Tharinger, D. J., Finn, S. E., Hersh, B., Wilkinson, A., Christopher, G. B., & Tran, A. (2008). Assessment feedback with parents and preadolescent children: A collaborative approach. *Professional psychology: Research and practice*, *39*(6), 600.

Thompson, L. & Thompson, M. (1988). Neurofeedback combined with training in metacognitive strategies: Effectiveness in students with ADD. *Applied Psychophysiology and Biofedback.* 23 (4) 243–63.

Thompson, S. (1997) *The Source for Nonverbal Learning Disorders*. East Moline, IL LinguiSystems Inc.

Tincani, M., Travers, J. C., & Boutot, A. (2009). Race, Culture, and Autism Spectrum Disorder: Understanding the role of diversity in successful educational interventions. *Research and Practice for Persons With Severe Disabilities*, *34*(3–4), 81–90. https://doi.org/10.2511/rpsd.34.3-4.81

Torres, K., Jaafar, I. & Statti, A. (2021). Addressing COVID Slide: How the Pandemic May Impact Future Learners. In E. Langran & D. Rutledge (Eds.), Proceedings of SITE Interactive Conference (pp. 274–277). Online, United States: Association for the Advancement of Computing in Education (AACE). Retrieved August 18, 2022 from https://www.learntechlib.org/primary/p/220202/.

Trammel, J., & Hathaway, M. (2007). Help seeking patents in college students with disabilities. *Journal of Postsecondary Education and Disability*, 20 (1) 5–15.

Trent, M., Dooley, D. G., & Dougé, J. (2019). The impact of racism on child and adolescent health. *Pediatrics*, *144*(2). https://doi.org/10.1542/peds.2019-1765

Tse, Y. J., McCarty, C. A., Stoep, A. V., & Myers, K. M. (2015). Teletherapy delivery of caregiver behavior training for children with attention-deficit hyperactivity disorder. *Telemedicine journal and e-health; the official journal of the American Telemedicine Association*, *21*(6), 451–458. https://doi.org/10.1089/tmj.2014.0132

Turan, S., & Eray, Ş. (2021). Impact of the pandemic on the mental health of children and clinical practice in Turkey: a narrative review with recommendations. *Scandinavian journal of child and adolescent psychiatry and psychology*, *9*, 160–162. https://doi.org/10.21307/sjcapp-2021-017

Valås, H. (2001). Learned Helplessness and Psychological Adjustment II: Effects of learning disabilities and low achievement. *Scandinavian Journal of Educational Research*, 45:2, 101–114. DOI: 10.1080/00313830120052705

Valle et al. (2010). The disability closet: Teachers with learning disabilities evaluate the risks and benefits of "coming out." *Equity & Excellence in Education,* 37: 1, 4–17.

Vallecorsa, A., DeBettencourt, L. U., & Zigmond, N. (2000). *Students with Mild Disabilities in General Education Settings: A Guide for Special Educators*. Prentice Hall.

Vaughn, S., LaGreca, A. (1993) *Social skills training: why, who, what and how in Learning Disabilities: Best Practices for Professionals*. Andover Medical Publishers, Boston MA.

Vidyasagar, T. R., & Pammer, K. (2010). Dyslexia: A deficit in visuo-spatial attention, not in phonological processing. *Trends in Cognitive Sciences*, *14*(2), 57–63. https://doi.org/10.1016/j.tics.2009.12.003

Vizard, T., Sadler, K. &, Ford, T. (2020) Mental Health of Children and young people in England. *Health and Social Care Information Center*

Vogel, S. A. (1987). Issues and Concerns in LD college programming. In DJ Johnson & J. W. Blalock (Eds.), *Adults with Learning Disabilities: Clinical Studies* (pp.258–276). Orlando, FL: Grune & Stratton.

Wachtel, P. L. (1993). *Therapeutic communication: Principles and effective practice.* Guilford Press.

Wachtel, P. L., & Messer, S. B. (1997). *Theories of psychotherapy: Origins and evolution.* American Psychological Association. https://doi.org/10.1037/10239-000

Waite, M. C., Theodoros, D. G., Russell, T. G., & Cahill, L. M. (2010). Internet-based telehealth assessment of language using the CELF-4. *Language, speech, and hearing services in schools,* 41(4), 445–458. https://doi.org/10.1044/0161-1461(2009/08-0131)

Waite, P., Pearcey, S., Shum, A., Raw, J., Patalay, P., & Creswell, C. (2021). How did the mental health symptoms of children and adolescents change over early lockdown during the COVID-19 pandemic in the UK?. *JCPP advances*, *1*(1), e12009. https://doi.org/10.1111/jcv2.12009

Waxmonsky, J. G., Waschbusch, D. A., Belin, P. J., Li, T., Babocsai, L., Humphery, H., Parizeau, M. E., Babinski, D. E., Hoffman, M. T., Haak, J. L., Mazzant, J. R., Fabiano, G. A., Pettit, J. W., Fallahazad, N., & Pelham, W. E. (2016). A randomized clinical trial of an integrative group therapy for children with severe mood dysregulation. *Journal of the American Academy of Child and Adolescent Psychiatry, 55*(3), 196–207. https://doi.org/10.1016/j.jaac.2015.12.011

Wechsler, D. (2009). *Wechsler Memory Scale–Fourth Edition*. New York: Pearson.

Wechsler, D. (2014) *The Wechsler Intelligence Scale for Children-Fifth Edition.* New York: the Psychological Corporation.

Wechsler, D. (2020) *Wechsler Individual Achievement Test (WIAT-4) (4th Ed)* San Antonio, TX: Pearson.

Westervelt, H. J., Brown, L. B., Tremont, G., Javorsky, D. J., & Stern, R. A. (2007). Patient and family perceptions of the neuropsychological evaluation: how are we doing? *The Clinical Neuropsychologist, 21*(2), 263–273.

White, S. W., Albano, A. M., Johnson, C. R., Kasari, C., Ollendick, T., Klin, A., Oswald, D., & Scahill, L. (2010). Development of a cognitive-behavioral intervention program to treat anxiety and social deficits in teens with high-functioning autism. *Clinical child and family psychology review, 13*(1), 77–90. https://doi.org/10.1007/s10567-009-0062-3

White, S. W., Stoppelbein, L., Scott, H., & Spain, D. (2021). It took a pandemic: Perspectives on impact, stress, and telehealth from caregivers of people with autism. *Research in developmental disabilities, 113*, 103938. https://doi.org/10.1016/j.ridd.2021.103938

White, S. W., Oswald, D., Ollendick, T., Scahill, L. (2009). Anxiety in children and adolescents with autism spectrum disorders. *Clinical Psychology Review*, Volume 29, Issue 1.

Winnicott, D. W. (1960). The True and False Self. In *The Maturational Process and Facilitating Environment* (pp. 140–152). New York, NY: International Universities Press.

Wong, A. W., & Landes, S. D. (2021). Expanding Understanding of Racial-Ethnic Differences in ADHD Prevalence Rates among Children to Include Asians and Alaskan Natives/American Indians. *Journal of Attention Disorders, 26*(5), 747–754. https://doi.org/10.1177/10870547211027932

Wood, C. L., Kelley, K. R., Test, D. W., & Fowler, C. H. (2010). Comparing audio-supported text and explicit instruction on students' knowledge of accommodations, rights and responsibilities. *Career Development For Exceptional Individuals* 33, 115–124.

Wyler, H., Liebrenz, M., Ajdacic-Gross, V., Seifritz, E., Young, S., Burger, P., & Buadze, A. (2021). Treatment provision for adults with ADHD during the COVID-19 pandemic: An exploratory study on patient and therapist experience with on-site sessions using face masks vs. Telepsychiatric Sessions. *BMC Psychiatry, 21*(1). https://doi.org/10.1186/s12888-021-03236-9

Xiang, M., Zhang, Z., & Kuwahara, K. (2020). Impact of COVID-19 pandemic on children and adolescents' lifestyle behavior larger than expected. *Progress in cardiovascular diseases, 63*(4), 531–532. https://doi.org/10.1016/j.pcad.2020.04.013

Xie, Y., Dixon, J. F., Yee, O. M., Zhang, J., Chen, Y. A., DeAngelo, S., Yellowlees, P., Hendren, R., & Schweitzer, J. B. (2013). A study on the effectiveness of videoconferencing on teaching parent training skills to parents of children with ADHD. *Telemedicine and E-Health, 19*(3), 192–199. https://doi.org/10.1089/tmj.2012.0108

Xu, C., Reid, R., & Steckelberg, A. (2002). Technology Applications for Children with ADHD: Assessing the Empirical Support. *Education and Treatment of Children, 25*(2), 224–248. http://www.jstor.org/stable/42900528

Yale School of Medicine (2017). The Yale Center for Dyslexia and Creativity *The Truth About Accommodations* http://dyslexia.yale.edu

Yell, M. L., Katsiyannis, A., Ryan, J. B., McDuffie, K. A., & Mattocks, L. (2008) Ensure compliance with the Individuals with Disabilities Education Improvement Act of 2004.Interventions *in School and Clinic* 44 (1) 45–51.

Yirmiya, N. & Sigman, M. (1991). High functioning individuals with autism: Diagnosis, empirical findings, and theoretical issues. *Clinical Psychology Review,* 11, 669–683.

Yngve, M., Lidström, H., Ekbladh, E., & Hemmingsson, H. (2018). Which students need accommodations the most, and to what extent are their needs met by regular upper secondary school? A cross-sectional study among students with special educational needs. *European Journal of Special Needs Education*, *34*(3), 327–341. https://doi.org/10.1080/08856257.2018.1501966

Yuan, N., Pevnick, J. M., Botting, P. G., Elad, Y., Miller, S. J., Cheng, S., & Ebinger, J. E. (2021). Patient use and clinical practice patterns of remote cardiology clinic visits in the era of COVID-19. *JAMA Network Open*, *4*(4). https://doi.org/10.1001/jamanetworkopen.2021.4157

Zablotsky, B., Bradshaw, C. P., Anderson, C., & Law, P. A. (2013). The association between bullying and the psychological functioning of children with autism spectrum disorders. *Journal of developmental and behavioral pediatrics; JDBP*, *34*(1), 1–8. https://doi.org/10.1097/DBP.0b013e31827a7c3a

Zaragoza, N., Vaughn, S., & Mcintosh, R. (1991). Social Skills Interventions and Children with Behavior Problems: A Review. *Behavioral Disorders*, *16*(4), 260–275. https://doi.org/10.1177/019874299101600407

Zhang, D., & Benz, M. R. (2017). Enhancing self-determination of culturally diverse students with disabilities: Current status and Future Directions. *Focus on Exceptional Children*, *38*(9). https://doi.org/10.17161/foec.v38i9.6823

Zhou, X., Snoswell, C. L., Harding, L. E., Bambling, M., Edirippulige, S., Bai, X., & Smith, A. C. (2020). The Role of Telehealth in Reducing the Mental Health Burden from COVID-19. *Telemedicine journal and e-health; the official journal of the American Telemedicine Association*, *26*(4), 377–379. https://doi.org/10.1089/tmj.2020.0068

Zylowska, L., Ackerman, D. L., Yang, M. H., Futrell, J. L., Horton, N. L., Hale, T. S., Pataki, C., & Smalley, S. L. (2007). Mindfulness meditation training in adults and adolescents with ADHD. *Journal of Attention Disorders*, *11*(6), 737–746. https://doi.org/10.1177/1087054707308502

Index

Page numbers in italics refer to boxes and tables.

About the Author

Dr. Nechama Sorscher is a clinical psychologist and neuropsychologist who maintains a private practice on New York City's Upper West Side, specializing in assessing and treating patients with learning and attention difficulties. Dr. Sorscher graduated with a PhD in Clinical Psychology from Adelphi University and has a Certificate in Psychotherapy and Psychoanalysis from NYU's Postdoctoral Program. She has published scholarly articles and book chapters on learning and attention difficulties as well as on trauma and child development. Additionally, Dr. Sorscher supervises and teaches psychological assessment at the William Alanson White Institute. She enjoys conducting individual and group psychotherapy, and regularly provides parent guidance and school consultations related to LD and behavioral functioning.

Made in the USA
Monee, IL
13 September 2026

62975272R00125